THE MIND AND ITS BODY

Founded by C. K. Ogden

The International Library of Psychology

GENERAL PSYCHOLOGY
In 38 Volumes

I	The Neurosis of Man	*Burrow*
II	Creative Imagination	*Downey*
III	The Caveman Within Us	*Fielding*
IV	Men and their Motives	*Flugel*
V	The Mind in Sleep	*Fortune*
VI	The Mind and its Body	*Fox*
VII	Practical Psychology	*Fox*
VIII	Man for Himself	*Fromm*
IX	The Law Within	*Fuller*
X	The Nature of Laughter	*Gregory*
XI	Readings in General Psychology	*Halmos et al*
XII	The Psychologist at Work	*Harrower*
XIII	The Psychology of Philosophers	*Herzberg*
XIV	Emotion	*Hillman*
XV	The Foundations of Common Sense	*Isaacs*
XVI	The Psychology of Consciousness	*King*
XVII	The Sciences of Man in the Making	*Kirkpatrick*
XVIII	The Person in Psychology	*Lafitte*
XIX	Man's Unconscious Passion	*Lay*
XX	Psychological and Biological Foundations of Dream-Interpretation	*Lowy*
XXI	Nervous Disorders and Character	*Mckenzie*
XXII	An Historical Introduction to Modern Psychology	*Murphy*
XXIII	Modern Theories of the Unconscious	*Northridge*
XXIV	The A B C of Psychology	*Ogden*
XXV	The Psychology of Thought and Feeling	*Platt*
XXVI	Introductory Psychology	*Price-Williams*
XXVII	Empirical Foundations of Psychology	*Pronko et al*
XXVIII	Psychotherapy	*Schilder*
XXIX	The Psychology of Time	*Sturt*
XXX	The Origins of Love and Hate	*Suttie*
XXXI	Art and the Unconscious	*Thorburn*
XXXII	The Elements of Psychology	*Thorndike*
XXXIII	Telepathy and Clairvoyance	*Tischner*
XXXIV	Human Psychology as Seen Through the Dream	*Turner*
XXXV	The Psychology of Self-Conciousness	*Turner*
XXXVI	The Psychology of Economics	*Weisskopf*
XXXVII	The Measurement of Emotion	*Whately Smith*
XXXVIII	How to be Happy Though Human	*Wolfe*

THE MIND AND ITS BODY

The Foundations of Psychology

CHARLES FOX

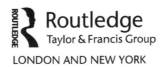

LONDON AND NEW YORK

First published in 1931 by
Kegan Paul, Trench, Trubner & Co., Ltd.
2 Park Square, Milton Park, Abingdon, Oxfordshire OX14 4RN
711 Third Avenue, New York, NY 10017

First issued in paperback 2014

Routledge is an imprint of the Taylor and Francis Group, an informa business

The publishers have made every effort to contact authors/copyright holders
of the works reprinted in the *International Library of Psychology*.
This has not been possible in every case, however, and we would
welcome correspondence from those individuals/companies
we have been unable to trace.

These reprints are taken from original copies of each book. In many cases
the condition of these originals is not perfect. The publisher has gone to
great lengths to ensure the quality of these reprints, but wishes to point
out that certain characteristics of the original copies will, of necessity, be
apparent in reprints thereof.

British Library Cataloguing in Publication Data
A CIP catalogue record for this book
is available from the British Library

The Mind and its Body
ISBN 978-0415-21018-8
General Psychology: 38 Volumes
ISBN 0415-21129-8
The International Library of Psychology: 204 Volumes
ISBN 0415-19132-7

ISBN 13: 978-1-138-87524-1 (pbk)
ISBN 13: 978-0-415-21018-8 (hbk)

TO
MY MOTHER

CONTENTS

*The figures in brackets in the text indicate the
References at the end of the book.*

PAGE

PREFACE xi

THE ARGUMENT 1

CHAP.

I. PSYCHOLOGICAL PHYSIOLOGY : THE THEORIES . 8

Descartes on the mechanical nature of vital processes—
Physiological dogmas (1) The cerebrum as the organ of
consciousness—(2) Sensations located in the cortex—
(3) Motor area the centre of voluntary movement—
(4) Point-to-point correspondence of brain and mind—
(5) Association dependent on association fibres—(6)
Memory a function of the brain—(7) The reflex theory—
Restitution of function—(8) Mental configuration mirrors
nerve configuration.

II. PSYCHOLOGICAL PHYSIOLOGY : THE FACTS . 26

Nerves do not convey sensations—The action current
and the all-or-none rule—Nervous impulses all alike—
Nerves do not convey messages—Chronaxy—Images do
not exist in the brain—Sensations not caused by impulses—
Conditioned reflexes—Meaning of ' stimulus '—The conditioned reflex is the law of association—Inhibition
essential to learning—Physiological and real animals.

III. PHYSIOLOGICAL PSYCHOLOGY : ANIMAL . . 52

Hartley on nerve function—Pathways or traces in
nervous system—Method of studying brain functions—
Equipotentiality of brain areas—Learning a function of
quantity of brain tissue—No point-to-point correspondence
of brain and mind—Cognition has no neural correlate—
Conditions of restitution of function are mental not neural—
No fixed association paths in the brain—The theory of
reflex action examined.

IV. PHYSIOLOGICAL PSYCHOLOGY : HUMAN . . 77

Discovery of aphasia—The invention of nerve centres—
Diagram makers—Hughlings-Jackson on aphasia—Apraxia
and agnosia—These disorders not due to loss of images—
Erroneous reasons for localization of function—Aphasia
not a simple defect—Head's views on aphasia—Aphasia and
other defects due to psychological deficiencies—Centres are

variable—The functions of the brain misconceived—
Neglect of psychological factors—Function not dependent
on structure—Localization of function inconsistent with
sound biology—Aphasia is a symptom of a wider defect—
The dogmas of the first chapter all unfounded.

V. PSYCHOLOGY OF LANGUAGE 104

The psychological standpoint explained—How a child
acquires language—Roots of the language faculty—
Emotional expression—The social factor—Symbolic significance—The sound stream—Linguistic identities—Linguistic values—The complexity of language and origin of
values—Does language express racial differences—Primitive
language — Language and the mind-body problem —
Language entirely a psychical product.

VI. PSYCHOLOGY OF TEMPERAMENT . . . 130

The classical doctrine—Glands determining temperament
—Physiological effects of emotion—Psycho-galvanic reflex
—Nerves and temperament—Ribot's two types of personality—Adopted by James and elaborated by Jung—
Extraverts and introverts—Physique and temperament—
Cyclothymes and schizothymes — Temperament and
character—What is temperament and is it inborn—The
scientific doctrine of temperaments unsound—Temperament like personality an artistic conception.

VII. MENTAL ENERGY 152

Modern view of energy—Attempts to measure fatigue—
A fund of energy in psychology—Physiological energy—
No analogy between mental and physical energy—Modern
doctrine of energy more closely considered—Fatigue and
energy—Facts of life and doctrine of energy inconsistent—
The facts of fatigue as measured—Fatigue and rhythm—
Danger of physical analogies.

VIII. INSTINCT AND CUSTOM 176

Criteria of instincts—Human instincts enumerated by
James, by Thorndike and by McDougall—The concept of
instinct not applicable to human action—The parental
instincts—Infanticide almost universal—The sexual instincts—Instinct of curiosity—The acquisitive instinct and
its measurement—Instinct of pugnacity—The aleatory
instinct—Thinking as an instinct—Energy and instinct—
Structure determined by function—Instincts and faculty
psychology—Inborn appetites all blind—Fear not an
inborn drive—No instinctive forces—Impulsive power of
habit.

CHAP.   PAGE

IX. A GREAT ILLUSION 203

Mental imagery an illusion—Characteristics of illusions—
Sensations and images differ in nature—Eidetic images—
Images, hallucinations, dreams—Sensations not revivable—
Subjective states alone revivable—Analysis of perception—
Empathy—Hallucinations—Illusion of false recognition or
déjà vu—Purely mental states revivable—Images have the
characters of illusions and are mistaken for objective things.

X. EDUCATIONAL PSYCHOLOGY 224

History of doctrine of mental discipline—Experiments
on transfer of effects of training—Theory of the experiments
—No identical elements in different situations—Modern
experiments—Importance of principles and ideals—
Mechanical and enlightened practice—Values and ideals.

XI. MIND MATTER AND PHILOSOPHERS . . . 240

Two separate problems : matter and mind, body and
mind—Aristotle on mind and body—Descartes on mind
and matter—Aristotle again—Descartes on mind and
body—Mind and body *versus* mind and matter—William
James' views—Spinoza—Monadology of Leibniz—Biological views—Mind-body relation unique—Modern view
of matter—Organic nature of matter—Mind and matter in
different realms.

XII. MIND AND BODY 261

The instrumental relation—Living and dead tissue—
Mind and brain—Unity of organism and environment—
No one-to-one correspondence of mind and brain—Nature
of physical Time—Nature of perceptual Time—Perception
of space—Reflex nerve units an artifact—Conditioned
reflexes a misnomer—Perseveration—Mind controls body—
Emergent evolution—Immediate rapport with other minds
—Objects, not sensations, perceived—The subjective
standpoint—Mind-body relation unique—Four terms in
the relation—Freedom of the will—Immortality of the
soul.

REFERENCES 303

INDEX 311

PREFACE

I have long felt the urgency of investigating the relation of mind to body in the light of recent discoveries. Without them the discussion of the relation is rather empty. It soon became evident that the road to such an investigation was strewn with an enormous tangle of neurological, psychological and logical presuppositions which had to be cleared out of the way. If this were done, although the difficulties might not be solved we should, at all events, clearly see what the problem is. Many of the difficulties arise because we apparently live in very different worlds. Ordinary people pass their time in a populous universe inhabited by other people and surrounded by all the choir of heaven and furniture of the earth. Psychologists live in a duller world for they only meet sense-organs, bundles of naked instincts and emotions, sensations and images, and occasionally experience ideas. In the philosophical universe the only things encountered are coloured patches, jarring noises without music and other lonely sense-data, together with the pale spectres of abstract logic. But the physicists have the worst time of it, for in their world nothing moves and little happens ; there is neither light nor warmth, but only a shower of symbols in an atmosphere of probability.

I have chosen to live in a concrete psychological world ; only I seem to recognize around me minds, souls and other interesting inhabitants disporting themselves. They all seem to me to be doing things all the time, and as this cannot possibly be due to physical energy, which science assures me has no power to do anything, I assume naturally that they are endowed with spiritual energy. I know positively that these other people feel and think pretty much as I do, and as it is certain that this cannot be demonstrated by any process of reasoning I feel perfectly convinced that it is innately known to me. If priority in time were any evidence of the innateness of knowledge it would not be difficult to demonstrate that self-consciousness is the result of the consciousness of other selves; for that is the order in which the knowledge comes to me. Cogitant ergo sum expresses it, if only we omit the ergo.

Moving in a concrete psychological world has its dangers but it has the compensating advantage of enabling us to deal with significant problems. For example, when the problem of the freedom of the will is considered it frequently tails off into a discussion of what happens when a man moves a limb or his body. But what this has to do with the question is by no means evident, for no man in initiating a course of action ever thinks of the movements of his limbs, unless he is paralysed and cannot move them. The real concrete problem involved in the discussion is whether a person (not a will) can create his own motives. And similar considerations apply to our other psychological problems which are all, therefore, treated concretely in our argument.

It is hoped that the method of treatment and the topics discussed will appeal not only to psychologists but to all who are interested in the wider aspects of the science of life. In order to enable the reader to assimilate the large mass of detail dealt with in the book, without losing the thread of the discussion, the argument has been set out at the start. It will help matters if this argument is read afresh at the end of every chapter.

Anybody who treats of the relation of mind to body must be conscious of his debt to a large number of other workers in a variety of fields. I have preferred to acknowledge my indebtedness by naming these in the body of the book at places where their help has been used. I desire also to thank my friend Dr Emanuel Miller, the psychopathologist, for reading the first four chapters and not being shocked at the treatment therein.

CHARLES FOX.

Warkworth House,
    Cambridge,
    September 1931.

THE MIND AND ITS BODY

THE ARGUMENT

As the range of topics covered in this book is extensive and the details very numerous, it will be of assistance to summarize the argument so as to show the thread of connection between the various parts. The point of view from which the discussion is conducted is almost purely psychological. In the first four chapters the contributions of physiology to the mind-body problem are considered. No treatment of the problem which ignores the recent revolutionary discoveries in neurology can be considered adequate. It is shown, however, that there are a number of dogmas associated with nerve physiology, some consciously and others unconsciously, but nevertheless strongly believed in. They are so numerous and so closely interwoven with the fabric of the science that it is difficult to unravel them.

The three chief amongst these, from the point of view of the mind-body problem, are the following. First, it is firmly held that the reflex is the sole type of nervous activity, and every kind of nervous action is believed to be composed of simple reflex units. Closely allied to this there is a strong belief in a one-to-one correspondence between mental events and brain events. The third, and in some respects the most important, is the belief that the cerebral cortex is the organ of conscious life, or at all events is in some special sense connected with consciousness in a more intimate way than any other bodily organ. These dogmas are examined again in the final chapter in the light of all the preceding discussion in the book. The general conclusion arrived at is that, in considering the mind-body problem, all the explanatory concepts are purely psychological. Opinions contrary to this

A

date back to the seventeenth century and have been tradition-
ally handed down to us, but must be revised in the light of
present-day knowledge. For the facts on which these dogmas
are supposed to rest are either erroneous or erroneously
interpreted.

The examination of these beliefs starts with an investigation
of nervous activity, which is submitted to close analysis, since
it is usually assumed that such activity is the cause of or
a necessary precursor to all conscious activity. The recent
discoveries connected with the restitution of function after
cerebral injury are considered in detail ; and these are shown
to shake the foundations of the dogmas previously considered.
A whole chapter is devoted to the problem of aphasia, since
this is one of the few kinds of disorder associated with cerebral
injury in which it is possible to secure first-hand introspective
evidence. The nature and extent of loss of function, when
we are dealing with the lower animals, is largely a matter of
individual interpretation. In the case of aphasia we can,
however, control the interpretation by getting direct introspective confirmation, more especially when dealing with
highly educated patients. Even here caution is necessary, as
the language defects that the patient suffers from at any
time seem to depend upon the personality of the physician
examining him.

The consideration of aphasia naturally leads to an investigation of the psychology of language, which is usually dealt
with perfunctorily by psychologists. It is shown that this
topic can be tackled without any reference whatever to its
supposed physiological basis. All the concepts employed in
the discussion are purely psychological. Difficulties in the
interpretation of aphasia and kindred disorders arise from
treating it as a physiological phenomenon. It is suggested, in
the text, that aphasia is but a symptom of some more fundamental mental disorder which has not yet been adequately
investigated.

At this point the argument turns back once again to
physiological considerations and treats in detail a doctrine
of the relation of mind to body which has persisted since

classical antiquity, namely the doctrine of temperaments. This rests on the dogma that the mind, in some way, must mirror the bodily constitution. Though the doctrine in its pure form has been abandoned, attempts to resuscitate it on the basis of internal glandular secretions are very much in evidence to-day. The temperaments were once attributed to bodily humours and are so again, except that the humours have now become hormones. If the view that glands determine temperament is correct, there would seem to be little point in discussing the relation of mind to body on any other grounds, but it could be left to the biochemist, since he alone could determine the imbalance of internal glandular secretions and so estimate, in advance, what kind of temperament to expect. In the meantime, our argument shows that science does not know what temperament is, and it is therefore a trifle early to call in the biochemist to discover its physiological basis. Temperament, like the wider notion of personality, is, in fact, not a scientific concept at all, but an artistic one, and can only be properly dealt with from the artistic standpoint. We might as well attempt an analysis of personal charm as try to deal with temperamental differences by analytical scientific concepts.

A recent view of temperament is based on the opinion that a classification is possible by taking account of the fund of nervous energy at the disposal of different people, yielding a division into hypokinetic and hyperkinetic temperaments. And considerable use is made of this notion of nervous energy in a variety of psychological fields. However, a confusion is always apparent in such cases in the use of terms. Nervous energy is confusingly mixed up with mental energy, and more often still the two are equated. A detailed examination of the concept of mental energy is undertaken. It is shown that there is no analogy between the concepts of mental and physical energy and the equation is, therefore, unsound. In particular, it is shown that no explanation of mental fatigue has ever been given on the basis of mental or even nervous energy. And this is most surprising, seeing that it is mainly for this purpose that the concepts ought to be employed, if they are workable. A new theory of fatigue is elaborated in the text in which these notions are ignored.

The modern doctrine of instinct, however, makes abundant use of the notion of mental energy and, more especially, of an assumed fund of energy at the disposal of each person. At this stage of the argument, therefore, the question of instinct in human activity is taken up and critically examined. The sex instinct and the parental instincts, as being the two most powerful in human nature, are discussed fully, since it is assumed that what is found to be true of these must apply to all the so-called instincts. It is shown that the doctrine of instinct, as expounded by the best modern writers, is based on an illegitimate series of abstractions. As far as human activity, at any rate, is concerned it is impossible to divorce instinct from custom. If this is accepted, then it follows that there are no such things as unchangeable instincts in human nature ; and the notion that instincts are inborn must be abandoned. In their place we must assume that custom or habit is not only the great regulator of human action but provides its motive force.

So far the argument has been largely critical. From this point onwards it becomes increasingly constructive. The first step in the process is to get a correct notion of that most obscure of all psychological concepts, the mental image. Whilst the nature of sensations has led to an enormous amount of discussion, the corresponding literature of mental imagery is brief and hopelessly unsatisfying. Mental images are supposed to be rather badly taken photographic copies of sensations. The films on which the photographs are taken, usually conceived as the brain centres of the corresponding sensations, are so badly made that the images are faint and very sketchy. Yet, despite their sketchiness, images are supposed to be perceived in exactly the same psychological way as sensations. All this appears to me to be due to an illusion, the nature of which is fully investigated in the text. The argument shows that the stuff of mental images is of a totally different kind from sensations, being purely subjective. This makes it quite unnecessary to suppose that mental images are dependent on the same brain centres as their corresponding sensations; or even to assume that there is any necessity whatever for an underlying physiological basis for images. If this view is justified it cuts the ground away from the belief that the mind is completely dependent on the body.

The purely subjective nature of mental imagery leads on to a consideration of the nature of subjective activity in general. When this latter notion is analysed a fundamental disparity is revealed between such activity and all forms of bodily activity. For the former is of a general nature whilst the latter is purely specific. When a man trains the muscles of his wrist by using a golf club, it would be preposterous to enquire whether his hearing, for example, can be improved by this process. Nevertheless, our argument shows that this sort of generalized effect, so far from being absurd in the realm of mind, is a matter of daily occurrence. Plato was correct when he maintained that a man who had studied one subject was infinitely superior to a man who had not, with respect to the better apprehension of all other subjects. The only explanation I can offer for this, is that the notion of subjective activity presupposes a spiritual world from which the motive force is derived. So that what is impossible in the realm of nature is easily realized in the realm of ends.

At this stage of the argument an attempt is made to grapple with the problem of the relation of mind to body at close quarters. The views of those philosophers are considered who have had anything original or constructive to say on the subject. The psychological standpoint from which our whole survey has, so far, been conducted is temporarily abandoned; to be resumed later. First of all, two different problems are disentangled; that of the relation of matter to mind, and that of body to mind. Unless these two are kept apart, in thought, nothing but confusion can result; and in actual fact such confusion is rampant. Many philosophers have a most unreasonable passion for unity; which leads them to treat the two problems as one. The greatest of them, however, after constructing their unified universe out of very unpromising material, have a strong suspicion that there really are two problems, and an uneasy feeling that they have considered only one. This leads to a rift in the philosophic universe which it is desirable in the interests of clarity to prize open a little wider. There is, however, one method by which the philosophic situation may be saved and a unified system preserved. This we owe to Professor Whitehead who has overcome the difficulty, not by explaining organic life in terms of physics, but by showing that physics is only intelligible in terms of organism. Such a change of front, which had been partially anticipated by Leibniz, constitutes a very considerable advance in the consideration of the mind-body problem. Nevertheless, it is not completely satisfactory in that it refuses to accept the irreconcilable differences between the subjective and the objective aspects of existence.

In the last chapter all the threads of the argument are woven together, and the conclusions which our survey of the problem have suggested are definitely stated, and backed up by further evidence. Chief among these is the fact that no explanatory value whatever attaches to any concept derived from the external world of science when applied to the study of mind. On the other hand, the only concepts which can be intelligibly used in describing the biological activities of a living organism are all derived from mental events. A moment's reflection will suffice to convince anybody that this must be the case. For how can an epistemology derived from the physical world be adequate to explain mental events which, *ex hypothesi*, are ruled out at the beginning. But mental concepts by themselves are shown to be insufficient, and the problem of the relation of mind to body requires a further set of notions derived from the spiritual world, the realm of ends. A psychology without a soul is a soulless psychology.

When a problem, such as ours, has engaged the attention of so many acute minds through so many generations with such unsatisfying solutions, the suspicion arises that the problem has been incorrectly stated. It is as though mathematicians had been attempting to find a solution of a problem with too few equations as their data. Our argument shows that there are, in fact, four sets of terms in the mind-body problem, not two. When the two extra sets of terms are introduced, certain long-standing difficulties may be solved ; for instance the question of the freedom of the will may be tackled as a significant problem instead of a game in abstract logic. The argument closes with a suggestion, hinted at in an earlier chapter, of a psychological method of approaching the most vital aspect of the mind-body problem, the immortality of the soul.

CHAPTER I

PSYCHOLOGICAL PHYSIOLOGY—THE THEORIES

THE axioms of modern psychological physiology are mainly derived from the theories of Descartes (1596–1650) as set out more especially in his treatise *On Man* in which he maintained that all bodily activity, without exception, is to be explained on mechanical principles. The organism is simply a very complicated machine. Distilled from the blood and stored in the brain there was a subtle fluid, wholly unique but subject to physical laws, known as 'animal spirits'. He explained nervous action as being due to the passage of such animal spirits, or as we should now say of nervous impulses, along nerve fibres which he thought were minute tubes. External objects had the power of agitating these animal spirits, or as we should now say of stimulating the nerves, and causing them to move along the fibres so as to evoke sensation or movement. The animal spirits thus served to link mind and body.

Descartes drew a sharp distinction between mind whose essence was thinking and body whose essence was extension, thereby effecting a separation of body and mind which has persisted to the present time. The theory which was popular in his day was that the soul, while consciously performing voluntary acts, unconsciously controlled vital functions such as breathing, digestion, etc. This is the theory that Descartes set himself to combat. Vital functions were, for him, just as mechanical as the movements of clocks which are due to springs and wheels. He considered that animals were only skilful automata all of whose activities admit of a mechanical explanation.

He attempted to explain memory in the same mechanical way. The motion of the animal spirits along the nerve tubes had " the power of forming certain passages which remain open after the action has ceased, or which at all events if they close, leave a certain disposition in the small tubes by means of which they can be more easily opened again ; just as if one drags some needles across a piece of cloth the small holes so made would remain open, or if they closed they would leave traces in the stuff, which would cause them to open more easily on another occasion. And it must be noted that if some only of the holes were opened again, this alone would suffice to reopen the others, especially if they had been opened several times together. This shows how the recollection of one thing may be excited by another which has been previously imprinted at the same time in the memory. So when I see fire I remember the heat since I felt the heat on the previous occasion when I saw the fire ". (1) *

The final passage in his treatise gives a concise view of his general position. " I desire you to consider that all the functions which I have attributed to this machine, such as digestion, the beating of the heart and arteries, nutrition and growth, breathing, waking and sleep, the perception of colours, sounds, tastes, heat, and other such qualities by the external senses, the impression of their ideas in the organ of the *Sensus communis* and of imagination, the retention or impression of these ideas in memory, the internal motions of appetites and passions ; and finally the external movements of all the limbs, which follow so suitably as well from the action of objects presented to sense as from the passions and impressions which are found in the memory, that they imitate as perfectly as possible those of a real man,—I desire you to notice that these functions follow quite naturally in the machine from the arrangement of its organs, exactly as those of a clock, or other automaton, from that of its weights and wheels ; so that we must not conceive or explain them by any other vegetative or sensitive soul, or principle of motion and life, than its blood and its animal spirits." (2) Now, as man, unlike the lower animals, has a soul, it must be brought into touch with the body somewhere so as to receive impressions. This must

* Figures in brackets in the text indicate references at the end of the book.

obviously be in the brain, since all the nerves of sense converge there; but as most parts of the brain are double and the soul is a unity we must place it in the centre of the mass, in the pineal gland. It is interesting to note the assumption underlying this reasoning as it pervades a good deal of current physiology. The assumption is that the mind somehow mirrors the brain. If two parts of the brain are stimulated there must be two impressions on the mind, and so on. This is a dogma about which we shall have a good deal to say later on.

The view that biological phenomena of every kind can be adequately explained on mechanical principles has, thanks to the influence of Descartes, persisted up to the present day. As a methodological device for physiological research it has justified itself by its success, but as an explanation of living and conscious process it is untenable. The conception underlying this sort of explanation was that it was possible for the human mind completely to grasp the nature of reality by the aid of mechanical models, interpreted by mathematical symbols. It was assumed that, outside of these model mechanisms, there was nothing left in nature to explain. Modern physicists, however, are coming round to the belief that their science is concerned with the symbolism alone, and teaches us little concerning the nature of ultimate reality beyond the fact that it may be grasped by symbolic treatment. Again, it was believed that an understanding of the present configuration of the material systems was completely adequate to forecast their future behaviour. The future was predictable from the past and present, so that nothing new or unexpected could emerge.

This situation is pithily described by Professor A. S. Eddington (3) who says: " One of the greatest changes in physics between the nineteenth century and the present day has been the change in our ideal of scientific explanation. It was the boast of the Victorian physicist that he would not claim to understand a thing until he could make a model of it; and by a model he meant something constructed of levers, geared wheels, squirts, or other appliances familiar to an engineer. Nature in building the universe was supposed to be dependent on just the same resources as any human mechanic ; and when the physicist sought an explanation of phenomena his ear was straining to catch the hum of machinery. . . . Nowadays we do not encourage the engineer to build the world for us out of his material, but we turn to the mathematician to build it out of his material. Doubtless the mathematician is a loftier being than the engineer, but perhaps even he ought not to be entrusted with the Creation unreservedly. We are dealing in Physics with a symbolic world . . . but if we are to discern controlling laws of nature not dictated by the mind it would seem necessary to escape as far as possible from the cut-and-dried framework into which the mind is so ready to force everything that it experiences."

Since Descartes' time, and largely as a result of his speculations, certain beliefs regarding nerve physiology have imperceptibly grown up, and have been adopted by psychologists with the conviction that not only are they reasonable in themselves, but their utility in psychological theory has given them the status of irrefutably established axioms. Some of these assumptions are mere guesses, and all of them are of doubtful validity. Yet it is widely thought that they are the established results of accurate experiment or observation, and it is mainly for this reason that psychologists employ them without hesitation or examination. Much of what passes in psychology for a study of habit, instinct, memory, imagination, etc., is simply a restatement of these physiological postulates translated into psychological terminology. These beliefs will now be formulated and examined in order to estimate their validity for the study of mind.

The most comprehensive of these assumptions, more frequently implied than stated, is that the cerebrum is the organ of consciousness. The activity of the brain and more especially the functioning of its outer layer, the cerebral cortex, is assumed to be the one essential immediate bodily cause of all mental activity. As the behaviour of the higher animals is more intelligent than that of the lower, and as this is paralleled by a corresponding development of the cerebral cortex, which reaches its maximum complexity in man, the assumption is held to be justified. An arrested development of the cerebral cortex is always accompanied by idiocy. And an instance is known of an infant lacking a cerebrum who survived for a few years and who lay almost motionless all the time without displaying any signs indicating mental reaction. He could be taught nothing. (4) Such facts as these, combined with the observation that injury to the cerebrum results, for a time at any rate, in loss of mental function are taken to be sufficient proof of the above-named supposition. Some physiologists, indeed, go further and assert that mental activity and cerebral functioning are two modes of stating the same fact. But this is a metaphysical theory smuggled into science for which the physiologist, as such, can have no justification whatever.

A less comprehensive form of the postulate we are considering limits it to the assumption that the one immediate bodily cause of every sensation or mental image is the activity of some specific area of the cerebral cortex. Such areas, the stimulation of which is supposed to be the sole cause of specific sensations are called sensory areas. Several of such areas have been mapped out on the cortex. There is the visual area in the occipital region, the olfactory in the hippocampal convolutions, the auditory area in the temporal lobe, the tactual area in the central convolutions and so forth. All these are anatomical regions in which the neurons from the various sensory or receptive organs of the body ultimately terminate, or are projected after a greater or less number of nervous relays. If the visual area of the cortex in the occipital region of the cerebrum is destroyed blindness is said to ensue, even when the retina and the optic nerves are uninjured, and hence it is called cortical blindness. Again any injury which severs the nerve connection between a sense organ and the brain leads to the loss of the corresponding sensation. Thus, if the spinal cord is severed, sensation below the seat of injury is lost. Facts such as these are regarded as sufficient evidence for the postulate.

The sensory areas occupy but a fraction of the surface of the cerebral cortex. In the year 1870 it was discovered that movements of certain isolated muscle groups could be produced by the stimulation of certain regions of the cortex. Such regions are in the vicinity of the central sulcus of the cerebrum, occupying mainly the central convolution anterior to the sulcus. The electrical stimulation of any portion of this area is followed by contraction of a particular group of muscles on the opposite side of the body. Hence this area of the brain is called the motor area ; and was thenceforward assumed to be the organ of voluntary movement. The sensory and motor areas by no means exhaust the surface of the cerebrum, and since the major part of the convolutions is occupied by fibres which run between these areas, bringing them into anatomical connection, they are lumped together as association areas. Each sensory projection area, after receiving afferent fibres from the sense organs, sends out " association fibres " to other parts of the cortex, in such a way that all parts of the cerebrum are in intimate physiological connection with all other parts. We shall return to these association fibres later.

Now there is nothing, at first sight, improbable in the localization of such functions as specific sensations or movements in different cerebral areas. This is a matter that is open to proof by investigation. But what are we to say about the attempted localization of such an activity as attention ? Anatomists have discovered that one of the distinguishing features of a gorilla's brain as compared with that of a human being consists of a great increase in the cortical area in the prefrontal region, *i.e.* the most anterior region of the cortex. As this region lies behind the forehead which gives the human head its most distinctive shape as compared with apes, it seems a pity to relegate such an area merely to the low grade function of association. Accordingly an important activity has been assigned to it. Thus Professor G. Elliot Smith (5), after explaining how the sense of vision becomes more differentiated and united with more delicate movements when arboreal life arose during the course of evolution, proceeds : " Such habits not only tended to develop the motor cortex itself, trained the tactile and kinæsthetic senses, and linked up their cortical areas in bonds of more intimate association with the visual cortex, but they stimulated the process of specialization within or alongside the motor cortex of a mechanism for regulating the action of that cortex itself. Thus arose an *organ of attention* (italics mine) which co-ordinated with the activities of the whole neopallium so as the more efficiently to regulate the various centres controlling the muscles of the whole body. . . . There was evolved from the motor area itself, in the form of an outgrowth placed at first immediately in front of it, a formation that attains much larger dimensions and a greater specialization of structure in the Primates than in any other Order. It is the germ of the great prefrontal area of the human brain which is *said to be concerned with attention* (italics still mine, but who said it ?) and the general orderly co-ordination of psychic processes. This area, in far greater measure than any other part of the brain, deserves of being regarded as the seat of the higher mental faculties and the crowning glory and distinction of the human fabric."

But surely such an important organ deserves a better office than to safeguard the old faculty psychology. Psychologists have long since ceased to believe in a separate faculty of attention. No doubt some faculties such as memory, imagination, etc., still carry on a precarious existence. If the higher mental faculties require a separate organ there is no place for an organ of attention. For attention is the kernel of *every* mental activity, high or low. A mental act without attention is a contradiction. To try to discover what a mental act without attention would be like is, as James somewhere says, to try to discover what the darkness looks like by switching on the light. It is a naïve psychology which first presupposes certain mental faculties and then adds to them a faculty of attention. Just as though a physiologist were to expect to find two sets of nerves, one to account for breathing and the other for taking in and expelling air.

Closely allied with the assumptions we have considered there is a postulate which has played a great part in the diagnosis of various disorders, such as aphasia. Just as there are certain areas of the cortex subserving vision, hearing, etc., so there are supposed to be certain collections of nerve cells with more complicated functions. Such collections are called

' centres ', and the best known of these is the centre of speech. The motor speech centre is located in the frontal lobe, and was originally placed there because an injury to certain convolutions in that region was associated with a loss of the ability to utter words. But all acquired capacities, such as reading and writing, are also supposed to develop their own centres. Each such centre, or collection of physiologically united cells, is thought to preside over its corresponding function, to initiate, control, and regulate it. Such centres are located not only in the cerebral cortex but also in sub-cortical regions. We may summarize this conception of centres by saying that there is supposed to be a point-to-point correspondence between brain structure and psychological functioning. This dogma of a correspondence is so firmly held by physiologists that psychologists have taken it over completely, and their discussions of the mind-body problem always assume it, as a matter of course. The important position assumed by this dogma justifies a minute examination, which will be undertaken later.

The theory of centres, by itself, is obviously inadequate to account for biological functioning even at the spinal level. Thus when the limbs of a decerebrate animal are stimulated we do not get isolated movements, but regularly co-ordinated series of movements. And it is this fact of co-ordination which is the distinguishing feature of living activity. Hence it is assumed that there must be " co-ordination centres " which inhibit or activate a whole muscular system so as to produce harmonious action. And it is assumed that such centres occur in large numbers in the cortex.

Professor H. Piéron in his brief but penetrating account of the nervous system (6) says, " it is the existence of these co-ordinating centres which is of primary importance in nervous functioning, and particularly in cerebral functioning." Now *pari passu* with the development of the brain in the evolutionary scale, and more especially with the growth of the cortex, there is a subordination and control of reflex movements. This is interpreted to mean that the nervous system is organized in levels whereby centres at a higher level control those at a lower level, in a sort of hierarchy. Piéron compares this work with the organization of a modern business house with co-ordinating and controlling officials on different floors. " Let us assume that there are four or five floors, the most complete organization is on the top. . . . When information arrives it is received by an agent in the office below, who transmits it to a connecting agent of his office, and also to the receiving agent in the office above, who likewise sends it on until it reaches the highest floor. Certain messages require a simple immediate response, indicated by the connecting agent below to his transmitting employees, but others necessitate a more complex elaboration. . . . The news is transmitted upwards from floor to floor and [if the intermediate agents are prevented from acting by their superiors] is considerably elaborated in the light of information already received, at the same time or later, by various receiving agents in the lowest floor ; and the order will then be communicated, directly this time and without delay at the intermediate floors, to the transmitting agents below, who are alone in communication with the outside world."

This ingenious comparison is thought to represent what actually occurs in the nervous system at the various coordinating centres at different levels. As however messages, news and orders all require interpretation by minds ; unless we are to assume that there are a number of minor minds all distributed over the nervous system with major minds at the top, it is perhaps better to change the simile and compare the nervous organization to an elaborate telephone exchange worked entirely on the automatic system with no minds at all anywhere in the system, except perhaps the engineer who thought it all out.

But, clever as this comparison is in subsuming the facts of nervous functioning, we must not be misled into supposing that the facts are only capable of this one interpretation. For Dr Henry Head has put forward a view which is equally capable of explaining the facts and has the merit of making less elaborate assumptions. (7) On the principle of Occam's razor, whereby an explanation with less elaboration is to be preferred to one with more assumptions, we may prefer this until a simpler comes to replace it. According to this view it is only necessary to adopt the one concept of *vigilance*. Thus suppose a man's spinal column is seriously injured, his lower limbs become flaccid, and reflexes are abolished. As the shock passes away the reflexes reappear and the nerves become so excitable that a slight stimulus will produce widespread and energetic action, the so-called mass-reflex; stimulation of any area may produce reflexes in widely separated parts, so that for instance tickling the foot may produce emptying of the bladder. If the patient develops fever he reverts to his original inert state again but on recovery the mass-reflex reappears. The shock of the injury has, as it were, brought about a low state of vitality which on passing away uncovers a high state of vigilance of the nervous system; higher than normal in fact, since the inhibitions of the intact nervous system are removed.

An intact nervous system does not necessarily mean increased excitability, but it does mean a more highly adapted response. Any injury to the system has an initial tendency to lower vitality and thus to depress this vigilance; for a time at any rate. All the facts of physiology, discovered by experiment or accidental lesions in different regions of the nervous system, may be interpreted in terms of a lowered state of vitality, leading to changed vigilance in different parts of the system. They can be accounted for, in other words, by a single concept, instead of a hierarchy of centres, some acting singly and others co-ordinating them. This, of course, does not settle the matter, for another concept may be found, somewhat less anthromorphic than the concept of vigilance.

So far all the postulates considered have had a more or less definite basis of observed physiological fact or experiment. We now enter the region of assumptions wherein the physiological data of observation are very meagre, or non-existent; and where the observations are psychological but are clothed in physiological terminology. The law of the association of ideas can be traced back to Aristotle and is founded on introspection. Stated very roughly, it means that, when a

B

series of ideas have been attended to in a certain order, the
subsequent arousal of the first member of the series leads to
the serial revival of the other members. This is interpreted
to mean, physiologically, that when on some occasion two
or more centres have been in action together, or in immediate
succession, a subsequent stimulation of one of the centres
will arouse the others to activity. As the centres in the brain
are joined by association fibres it is supposed to be easy to
see how the stimulation of one can awaken the others. It
must be remembered, however, that the function of such
pathways between centres is purely hypothetical. It rests on
the assumption that there must be some bond of union between
ideas which are associated, and that these bonds require a
nervous path. In other words the purely psychological law
of association is supposed to need connecting fibres, and is
therefore conveniently provided with them. To call such
fibres ' association fibres ' and to assume that they must,
therefore, be connected with the ' association of ideas ' is
merely a play upon words.

The process is assumed to work as follows. When a baby
sees a light a nervous current is supposed to run from the
lower visual centres to the motor area prompting him fatally
to push his finger into the flame, by a purely reflex act. This
is followed by pain, and the current now runs from the pain
centre to the motor area, leading to reflex withdrawal of the
finger. Now these reflex currents are supposed not only to
flow downwards to the muscles but also upwards to the
cortex ; and by this convenient arrangement the sight of the
flame, the pain in the finger, and the withdrawal, all three
leave traces of themselves in the cerebral centres. The
subsequent appearance of the flame arouses the image of the
painful sensation together with the idea of withdrawal. All
this is the crude psychology of a bygone age and the physiology
is equally primitive. For it is clear that the sight of the flame
ought on the second occasion to stimulate the pushing of the
finger into it, for a ' pathway ' has been left between these
centres. In order to get over the difficulty it is supposed
that the nervous processes in the cortical centres are of

greater strength than those in the lower centres ; and other equally arbitrary assumptions are made to get the scheme to work. It was found necessary to short-circuit the nervous currents in various ways so as to get them to run in the required paths. This elaborate scheme was once provided by the Austrian anatomist Meynert (8) and led to an era of diagram construction in which the nervous paths were carefully delineated. The scheme is now abandoned, but the diagrams, or their later copies, still survive. And the assumptions underlying the diagrams are still very much in evidence, though only tacitly approved.

There is but a short step from the explanation of the association of ideas by cortical paths to the explanation of memory in the same fashion. And the assumption that memory is a function of the cerebrum is the next postulate of psychological physiology. A violent blow on the head, or any other injury to the cortex, may lead to a permanent or temporary loss of memory, especially of the events immediately preceding the blow. Moreover, as we have seen, the various sensory areas are supposed to be the seats of different sensations. The cerebral hemispheres are accordingly said to be the seat of memory. When a sensation has been aroused by the activity of the appropriate area, a ' vestige ' of this is thought to be ' stored up ' in that area, very much in the way in which a gramophone record stores up sound. An external object produces a sensation by stimulating a sensory area, but when the same area is stimulated internally it arouses an image or an idea. This belief rests on the assumption that an image or an idea is simply a faint copy of a sensation. But there is no reason whatever to suppose that this is the case, and there is no psychological evidence to support it. Nobody has ever stimulated a sensory area by an internal process and produced an image ; and anybody who has experienced a mental image can assure himself that it is qualitatively different from any sort of sensation. Here, as with the former postulates, the belief rests on the determination to preserve a physiological substratum for mental life at any cost. It should be carefully noted, in this connection, that not only will a physical shock produce a loss of memory, but a purely mental shock, such as the sudden receipt of bad news will produce the same effect.

The next dogma that we shall consider really does, at first sight, appear to rest on physiological evidence, instead of being psychology distorted into hypothetical physiology. This is the assumption of the universality of reflex action, namely that every movement or other activity of the organism, or some part of it, is the necessary result of some stimulus, whose effect is reflected back to a muscle or gland ; the connection between the stimulus and the response being reflected through a fixed nervous pathway. Just as the push of an electric bell will inevitably cause the bell to ring when the cell is intact and the circuit unbroken, so a stimulus applied to an animal will call out the appropriate response. A bright light directed into the eye will cause the pupil to contract, independently of the will of the person and entirely without his knowledge. He will at the same time close his eye, and this he does equally reflexly but not necessarily unknowingly. This fatality or inevitability of reflex action is obviously bound up with the mechanical view of the functions of the body. If the mechanism of an automatic machine is in working order, dropping in a coin will inevitably yield the box of matches or cigarettes. In the same way the application of a stimulus to an organism will fatally produce the response, namely movement or glandular activity or other action. Hence another characteristic of a reflex is its predictability. This concept of reflex action is now applied not only to the activity of the spinal cord and lower parts of the brain, but to nervous action in general, including that of the cerebral cortex. There is supposed to be only one type of nervous action pervading the whole nervous system, the reflex type. The higher centres are thought to introduce no new modes of activity, but merely more and more complicated networks of connections. Such complications may lead to integration of nervous impulses, or to inhibition of activity, but the same type of action is said to persist. Reflex action is inconsistent with spontaneity, since it is dependent on some stimulus external to the reflex arc. Such lack of spontaneity, combined with the characteristic of fatality, would seem to imply a sharp division between reflex and voluntary action, unless the spontaneity of the latter is a delusion.

As this conception of reflex activity is so universally accepted it is desirable to get clear what modern physiology means by reflex action. (9) Many actions of animals are due to changes in the environment, which act as stimuli. The energy used up in the action is traceable to the potential energy in the chemical compounds in the animal's tissues, which is liberated by the stimulus in much the same way as a spark will cause an explosion. In unicellular organisms one and the same structure receives the stimulus, transmits a change from point to point and finally changes its form, or moves. But in higher organisms separate structures carry out the parts of the total change. Thus, if I turn my head in response to a sound, the auditory apparatus receives the stimulus, the auditory nerves convey an impulse to the central nervous system, and the impulse is reflected by other nerves to the muscles of the neck, which, by contracting, cause my head to move. So the reflex system comprises a receptor organ, a conductor which is always the nerves, and an effector organ such as a muscle or gland. In the living animal reflex activities are said to be co-ordinated, one with another, either simultaneously to form what is called a reflex pattern, or successively to make a succession of reflex patterns. Now it must never be forgotten that the co-ordination and integration are the primary facts of observation, and that the simple unit or reflex act is a pure abstraction which is invented to explain them. This convenient abstraction, whereby all nervous activity is explained as being due to the composition of simple reflex units, has been of the greatest assistance to the development of physiology, but has introduced incalculable confusion into psychology. The troubles which have arisen from the fact that cortical activity is considered to be merely reflex action will be considered later. In the meantime the general relation of consciousness to the brain may be mentioned.

If consciousness is the result of cortical functioning this

cannot be due, it is said, to any peculiar variety of nervous action foreign to the simplest reflex nervous process, but can only be due to the greater complexity of connections of the nervous paths. It is difficult to understand why a process, which is assumed to be entirely devoid of consciousness, acquires this property when it is multiplied or integrated. Two explanations have been offered of this perplexing phenomenon. Consciousness may be the invariable accompaniment of all nervous action, including that at the reflex level. If we take as the criterion of conscious activity the ability to pursue an end, with appropriate variations of means to that end, then it may be possible to suppose that consciousness accompanies reflex actions. For, if a noxious stimulus such as a prick is applied to the skin of a dog whose spinal cord is severed from the brain, the animal will try to remove the object by scratching with the foot of the same side. Should this be prevented it will make use of the opposite foot. Here we have a choice of means to accomplish a useful end, which in accordance with the above criterion makes reflex actions conscious.

If the above view is rejected, then we must fall back on the doctrine of emergent evolution according to which consciousness, which previously did not exist, suddenly emerges as a new fact at some higher nervous level. When a particular configuration of the nervous system develops, it carries with it a new feature of which there was no trace at an earlier stage. This view is taken by eminent philosophers, but it is difficult to see that it is more than a roundabout way of saying that we have no explanation whatever of conscious process, and that we cloak our ignorance by saying that it emerges from the void. It is quite possible that this is all we are justified in saying, and that we shall never be able to account for consciousness further than by assigning the conditions which precede its emergence. As far as the simplest conscious processes such as sensations are concerned, we certainly have no means of accounting for their emergence. All that we can do is to specify the set of nervous conditions which precede their arousal. The doctrine of emergent or creative evolution has such important bearings on the mind-body problem that it will be considered in detail later on, and from the purely psychological standpoint.

We have now enumerated the main postulates of psychological physiology and indicated the basis on which they rest. Before considering their validity in detail, it is desirable to call attention to one phenomenon, which has long been known and is difficult to reconcile with some of these postulates. We saw that the parts of the cortex most exactly studied, from the functional standpoint, are the motor areas. Each voluntary muscle is represented in the anterior central convolutions, in such a way that the stimulation of certain points produces movements of the opposite parts of the body ; for the nerve fibres traverse the medial line to the opposite parts of the nervous system. It was thought, for some time, that the various centres in the motor areas were sharply defined, that is to say that the stimulation of a restricted part of the right motor cortex (say) produced a contraction of the left thumb, whilst stimulation of another point contracted the eyelid and so on. But it has been found recently that successive stimulation of the same point of the motor area on different days produces movements of different parts ; and that sometimes flexion, and sometimes contraction, results from the stimulation of the same point. There appears to be no such fixity of function as has been supposed. As Dr Henry Head has pertinently observed " Provided the stimulus remains unchanged in strength and quality, an apparatus, working on purely mechanical principles, would continue to turn out identical products. This is notoriously not the case, even with the isolated spinal cord . . . no two successive excitations, however similar, are followed by the same result." The same stimulus may even inhibit an original reaction, or a new feature may appear, as when the stimulation of some point on the cortex which has produced contraction of the face at one time may suddenly yield flexion of the elbow. Such varying modes of response point to variations in vigilance of the same cortical point, and make the notion of reflex activity inapplicable to cortical action.

Again, when the whole of the motor cortex on one side of the body is destroyed, hemiplegia or paralysis of the opposite half of the body occurs, as we should expect. But the strange thing is that recovery from this condition happens sooner or later. The rate of recovery varies with the position of the animal in the evolutionary scale. In the case of rats the recovery is a matter of hours, in dogs it happens in a day or two and after a few weeks they are able to use their limbs on the paralysed side apparently as well as on the other side, though the latter are used by preference. With monkeys, apes and men the recovery takes longer but does nevertheless occur. After some months a monkey which has suffered from complete ablation of the motor areas on one side of the brain can use its voluntary muscles of the opposite side of the body so well that it is very difficult to detect any difference.

This phenomenon of restitution of function is obviously inconsistent with any rigorous view of localization of function in the brain or any supposition about definite ' centres ' subserving certain capacities. Two theories have been put forward to account for these inconvenient facts. According to one of them, when any cortical centre is destroyed, there is vicarious action of some other part of the cortex or of some lower centre. That is to say these other parts acquire new functions which they never had before, to meet the abnormal situation. If this is so, then it would appear that the functions of different parts of the brain are interchangeable. The second theory is that other cortical, or lower centres, resume functions that they have always had, but which are normally inhibited in the uninjured brain. The fact of inhibition is well established and will be studied later. In the meantime it is obvious that this theory, likewise, supposes that various parts of the cortex are functionally interchangeable, and that there can also be interchange of function between the cortex and lower centres. In any case we may conclude, that if either of these views is justified, it is very difficult to see how most of the postulates that were considered above can be maintained.

There is one further assumption of a general kind, which

is never expressly formulated, but is tacitly presupposed in psychological physiology. This is the view that the form, pattern or configuration of mental contents must somehow be mirrored in a corresponding pattern or configuration of brain processes. Thus, if I think of two things it is supposed that two cells must be involved. When I have two ideas, associated with one another, there must be an association fibre uniting two centres. That is to say, the complexity of the object of thought must be reproduced in a corresponding complexity of the brain processes ; and these latter must somehow reproduce the former pictorially. Again, since a mental image is supposed to be a faint copy of a sensation, it is assumed that the same brain process which causes a sensation must be taking place in a less intense manner to produce an image. The absurdity of supposing that if I think of a triangular object the underlying brain process must be itself triangular would, of course, not be countenanced. But the assumption we are considering is none the less absurd. There is no reason whatever to suppose, and there are good reasons for denying, that there is a point-to-point correspondence between brain processes and mental events. The atomic view of mental life, as consisting of a number of isolated elements, has long since been abandoned ; but brain events are separate and distinct occurrences. Consequently there can be no correspondence between them. It will be realized that the assumption, just considered, is a logical variant of the point-to-point correspondence theory between brain and mind, which we have already touched upon, but must consider more fully in a later chapter.

CHAPTER II

PSYCHOLOGICAL PHYSIOLOGY—THE FACTS

WE shall proceed to examine the assumptions previously enumerated in order to get some light on the relation of body to mind. This difficult problem has long been attacked on general metaphysical or psychological grounds but it seems desirable, at the start, to enquire what solution is suggested by physiological data. As it is obviously the nerves which put us in touch with the external world, and also with our own bodily organs, the first step is to get a correct notion of the nature of the nervous impulses underlying sensation and muscular action.

What is it that the nerves convey and the central nervous system registers? It is frequently implied that the optic nerve conveys sensations of light, the auditory sensations of hearing, and so forth. Sensations, as we know them, are supposed to be known to the nerves, and in some way travel along them. When a red patch of light, for example, is focussed on the retina it is assumed that the redness, in some mysterious fashion, travels up the optic nerve to the visual area of the brain where the sensation of red is registered. Stated in any such blunt fashion the assumption seems absurd, but nevertheless the belief and its implications are widely held. A little reflection will convince anyone that Professor G. F. Stout's view is the correct one. (1) " The sky is blue, but the sensation by which I apprehend the sky is a sensation *of* blue or *of* blueness. The road may be hot and fatiguing and the man hot and fatigued. His sensations, however, are not hot nor fatiguing. They are sensations of heat and fatigue. Similarly a sensation of sweetness is not itself sweet ". Despite this, which is obviously correct, it is supposed that when we listen to speech, for example, the words are conveyed to the speech areas of the brain, and recorded and stored there somewhat after the fashion of gramophone records. If it is objected that a gramophone record does not contain the words but only a series of corrugations or grooves, this is supposed to help the analogy ; since the brain centres are assumed to store up a similar series of configurations, reproducible under appropriate conditions. Whether this is so or not, and it will be examined later, it is evident that there is no justification for believing that the nervous system can either convey a sensation or store an image. What then is it that the nerves convey ?

Now a nerve fibre is the prolongation of a nerve cell and consists of a thread of protoplasm usually surrounded by an insulating fatty sheath. Such fibres, in man, are not more than a hundredth of a millimetre in diameter, but are sometimes more than a metre long. A nerve trunk, such as the sciatic, will contain several thousand of such fibres, some of them conveying centripetal and others centrifugal impulses, *i.e.* to or from the central nervous system. Any disturbance, such as an electric current, or a mechanical shock, or other change which will arouse the nerve to activity, is called a stimulus. As an electrical stimulus can be accurately measured and graded, our most exact physiological knowledge of nervous activity is derived from electrical stimulation. When a fibre is stimulated a wave of negative potential passes along it ; that is to say, the points of the fibre successively reached by the impulse become electrically negative to the rest of the nerve. Such a succession of disturbances, indicated by the wave of negative potential, has received the name of the ' action current ' of the nerve fibre, and is a very sensitive method of detecting the nervous impulse. In human nerves these impulses travel at the rate of a hundred metres per second. The highest magnification of such impulses, such as that produced by a five-thousand-fold valve amplifier, shews no difference whatever between centripetal and centrifugal impulses, *i.e.* between those passing along so-called sensory or motor fibres. Whilst the action current is passing, the nerve is completely inexcitable to a second stimulus ; so that the action is intermittent, and a constant stimulus must produce a series of discrete impulses.

It has been demonstrated by Dr E. D. Adrian that the intensity of the impulse *in a single nerve fibre* cannot be varied by changing the strength of the stimulus. (2)   Either the stimulus produces an impulse of given strength, or it is too weak to have any effect at all.   The sole effect of increasing the strength of the stimulus is to bring more fibres of the nerve trunk into play ; but the intensity of each impulse is not changed.   This is known as the ' all or none ' rule, and shews that the nervous impulse is a change which, for the time being, utilizes all the available resources of the nerve fibre. We may say, then, that a nervous impulse is an explosive change, determined by the conditions in the nerve itself, and making use of the potential energy stored in the resting fibres. It is very important to notice that the energy used in the explosion is derived from the substance of the fibre itself, and not from the stimulus.   Should the impulse ultimately reach a muscle the latter contracts, and the energy necessary to produce the contraction is derived from the chemical substances stored in the muscle ; the impulse acting like the trigger of a gun.   It is quite possible, by repeated stimulation of the nerve, to produce such a state of fatigue in the muscle that it is no longer able to contract ; nevertheless the impulses will still pass along the nerve.   This evidently shews that the energy is not transmitted from the nerve to the muscle.

The nature of centrifugal impulses in motor nerves has been studied for a long time, since the contraction of the muscles attached to the nerve provided a ready method of detecting their effects.   By availing ourselves of the enormous magnification produced by valve amplifiers, it has now been found possible to study the nature of centripetal impulses in sensory fibres.   By this means action currents have been observed in the auditory nerve of a rabbit in response to a sound, in the proprioceptor nerves of muscles when a limb is stretched, and in the excised optic nerve of a conger-eel when the eye was exposed to light.   No trace of any specific activity was found in the sensory nerve to correspond to the specificity of the particular sense organ. That is to say, the action current in the optic nerve does not differ fundamentally from that of the auditory nerve ; and neither differs from that found in the motor nerves. And the same ' all or none ' relation holds for sensory as for motor neurons. Dr Adrian, to whom we owe a good deal of our knowledge on this subject, sums up the experimental results by saying that " there are no radical differences between the impulses which produce the various modes of sensation ".

Imagine a physiologist from Mars who knew nothing about our sensations and wished to detect them and study their varieties. Guided by his colleagues on earth, and provided with the most powerful valve amplifiers, he traces the nerve impulse proceeding along the various nerves. The only distinctions he would notice between them might be certain differences in the time relations of the impulses ; nothing more. He would have no inkling of the fact that these impulses produced sensations ; still less that they produced different sensations according to the sense organ stimulated. He could not even tell whether an action current was on its way to awaken a sensation or arouse a muscular movement, since the only difference that he would detect between these would be that the one was centripetal and the other centrifugal. If he insisted on tracing the impulses further along the nerves to their central connections in the brain he would be no wiser. For the optic nerve is morphologically part of the brain, and consequently the connecting fibres in the brain must discharge impulses of the same kind as those found in the peripheral nerves, i.e. a series of intermittent impulses. No doubt a smoothing process of the volley of impulses occurs in some region of the brain, since it has been shown by Sherrington that in the spinal cord a brief series of centripetal impulses provokes a motor discharge of much more gradual onset, owing to the impulses being integrated and issuing in a final common centrifugal path. By analogy, therefore, our Martian physiologist would suspect that a smoothing process of a much more effective kind would occur somewhere in the brain ; and he would probably find this to be the case, since

the large number of connections found there would provide
an adequate anatomical basis for the smoothing.

If he were told, as he would have to be, for he would have
no means of discovering it for himself, that in the end a
sensation would emerge from the integrated impulses, and that
it would differ according to the particular set of nerves along
which the impulses travelled, he would regard it as a severe
tax on his credulity to believe this. Nevertheless, the most
careful research has failed to reveal any differences between
the nerve impulses in various sensory or motor fibres. As
Dr Adrian has said " the quality of the sensation seems to
depend upon the path which the impulses must travel, for
apart from this there is little to distinguish messages from
the different receptors ". Our Martian physiologist would,
of course, wonder how a difference in direction of the impulses
could distinguish a sight from a sound, and both from a pain
or a movement. But no one would be able to enlighten him.

As it is erroneous to say that the nerves convey sensations,
it is often asserted, as in the above quotation, that they carry
messages. Now, when a messenger conveys a message he
really does what he is asserted to do, that is communicates
a message either verbally, or in writing, or in some other
symbolic way. When a telegraph wire transmits a message,
what is sent across the wire is a series of currents, which,
being arranged in a variety of patterns, convey symbolically
a variety of meanings. But we have seen that the ' messages '
transmitted along the nerves are all of the same simple pattern.
They consist of a volley of impulses which are very much
alike whether they are destined to arouse sensations of light,
hearing, touch, pain, etc. Since the impulses are of the same
nature, and have no distinctive pattern, it is misleading to
speak of them by the name of messages. To call them by
this name conveys an implication for which there is no justification. If they were messages it would need a mind to decipher
them just as a telegraph operator is required to interpret
a code, but in our case the messages are always the same.
Even to call them signals goes too far, for signals must differ
if they are to have any significance, whereas nerve impulses

are all alike, so that the mind has to perform the mysterious operation of giving totally different meanings to signals which are all alike.

We have repeatedly referred to the path taken by a nervous impulse. Now the nervous system, and especially its central portion, presents an enormously complicated variety of possible paths ; and the question naturally arises as to how the impulses find their way through such an intricate network of directions. Along such a multiplicity of possible routes how is it that any specific direction can be maintained or repeated ? If an animal is poisoned by strychnine general convulsions occur in response to the slightest stimulus, *i.e.* an impulse set up anywhere runs over the whole central nervous system. Why does this not happen normally ? When a railway train approaches a junction its direction is determined by setting the points and shunting. And it is usually said that the rôle of the central nervous system is to shunt impulses along the appropriate paths. But how does the neuron play the part of a shunter ? This difficulty is usually ignored by treating the matter anthropomorphically : as though the neurons could decide to vary the resistance at their synapses at will.

Now L. Lapicque (3) has shewn that there is a physical basis for the restriction of the nervous impulses to certain directions. Neurons are not only anatomically distinct, but vary in specific conductivity. Each neuron, just like the different strings of a musical instrument, has its own periodicity. When an impulse has travelled along a certain neuron it ultimately reaches some synapsis or network of junctions with other neurons. The final direction of the impulse will be determined by the relative periodicities of the neighbouring fibres. The characteristic resonance, or time constant, of each nerve is called its chronaxy. If an electric current of constant intensity is suddenly passed through a nerve fibre connected to a muscle and continued indefinitely, the start of the current will provoke a contraction. Now, in accordance with the ' all or none ' rule a certain liminal intensity of the current will be necessary to cause a contraction, and below this intensity no effect will be produced. Such threshold of intensity for any particular nerve is called its rheobasis. If the duration of the current is progressively shortened, a time will come when no impulse is set up by the stimulus; and in order to provoke an impulse, with a current of very short duration, it will be necessary to augment its intensity. The minimum duration necessary to attain the threshold of excitability, with twice the rheobasic intensity, is taken to be the measure of the chronaxy of a nerve; and differs in different nerves. Thus, whilst the same ' all or none ' rule of excitability applies to every nerve fibre, there are enormous differences from one to another, depending on their chronaxies. When a neuron is stimulated the action current which travels along it will have its course into other neurons determined by their chronaxies. Each neuron, by virtue of its own time constant, acts as a sort of resonator picking up impulses from other isochronic neurons.

There is, however, a certain amount of irradiation when the exciting cause reaches greater intensities, bringing new fibres and new isochronisms into play. Moreover, as neurons are living structures their chronaxies can be considerably modified by various means, as by fatigue, toxic or other chemical agencies, as well as by increasing the intensity of the excitation. An important property of living tissue is its rapid modification resulting from its own activity, which is displayed in the well-known phenomenon of facilitation or habit. Tissues grow to the mode in which they are exercised. In this manner nervous activity tends to provide the conditions for future activity of the same kind. When, for any reason, one neuron has reacted to the impulse from another, the chronaxy of the former is modified in the direction of the latter. Such approximation of the time constants lasts for a considerable time but may gradually disappear, unless renewed by further activity. The nervous impulse, in other words, establishes the conditions for its own propagation. In this way a mechanism for shunting impulses through the complicated nervous system is provided. It is also reasonable to suppose that the chronaxies or time constants of different fibres are, to a large extent, determined by the activities of other parts of the nervous system. For it is a biological law that the functioning of every cell is dependent on that of all other cells in its environment. Seeing that all vital activity is regulated and co-ordinated activity, it is a mere abstraction to consider the action of an isolated fibre. What happens in one fibre is partly determined by what is occurring, or what has occurred, in all others : so that chronaxies are only relatively fixed. If we confine our view to artificial abstractions from life, such as the passage of an impulse along an isolated fibre, there is little to distinguish the living from the non-living. R. S. Lillie, for example, has shewn that an iron wire, first placed in strong nitric acid and then in a more dilute solution, is not attacked but maintains a passive state. When, however, it is ' stimulated ' by being touched with another piece of iron it shows the usual effervescent activity at that point. The ' impulse ' travels along its entire length and is even transmitted to another wire in contact with it, in a way which is a remarkably close copy of the transmission of an impulse in a nerve fibre.

It is conceivable that a model brain might be constructed in which all nerve tracts were made of iron wires and it would then be possible by ' stimulating ' the model to reproduce the impulses in all their complexity, and even to integrate and co-ordinate them. Since no sensation could ever emerge from such an artifact, it is clear that sensations are not conveyed by nerves, and that living tissue is an essential part of the physical basis of sensation. But the living nervous system simply provides the physiological conditions for the arousal of sensations ; whilst the existence of a mind is the essential condition, without which the nerves are powerless. In a similar way, it has been presumed, without any evidence, that a necessary condition for the arousal of mental images is the integrity of the nervous system, or certain parts thereof ; but it would be a soulless blunder to suppose that if this condition were fulfilled it would be sufficient, or that images can be, in any intelligible sense, stored in the brain. The two things, sensation and image, are exactly on a par in this respect.

c

The immediate bodily condition for a sensation is, then, a series of isochronous neurons beginning in a sense organ and ending in the brain. Any stimulation of the receptor portion of this series sends an impulse through the whole series and a sensation emerges. Thus, a pressure of the finger on the eyeball, by producing the necessary disturbance on the retina, leads to a series of impulses in the optic nerve and its isochronous neurons, and evokes a sensation of a coloured circle of light. Irritation of the exposed end of the sciatic nerve will provoke a sensation in an amputated leg. Now, it would be absurd to suppose that the coloured circles of light are pre-existent, and that we become aware of them when the eyeball is pressed, or that the sensations in the amputated limb exist and that the irritation transmits them, and makes us conscious of them. What exists in all these, and similar cases, is a nervous apparatus conveying a set of impulses, and a mind ready to respond to them, by virtue of what it has experienced before. It has been advisable to emphasize this, owing to certain beliefs which are widely countenanced by psychologists. When a mental image is aroused, it is believed that the image had a previous existence like the shades on the banks of Styx, and was waiting to be called back into the light of day. The psycho-analysts in particular give elaborate accounts of the antics of these shadowy images struggling to be free. This is about as reasonable as the belief that when I suffer from a hallucination, the hallucinatory appearance has been there all the time, struggling to emerge into my consciousness, and stepping in when it gets the chance.

What really happens in this case, is that a series of impulses have been set going in my sense organs and nerves, just in the same way as when I press my eyeball and see the circle of light. There was no pre-existing patch of colour in the one case, and there is no Stygian ghost in the other. Similarly when a mental image is aroused it comes into existence when it is perceived. It has often been supposed that the system of isochronous neurons, which is the condition for a sensation, may, when stimulated internally, give rise to a hallucination or an image. There is no positive evidence for this, which is merely suggested by the supposed similarities between sensations and images. But, as we shall see in a later chapter, an image is qualitatively different from a sensation, is composed of different material and cannot therefore depend on nervous conditions ; certainly not on nervous conditions alone. The important point is that there is no reason whatever to assume the existence of images in some dim region prior to their evocation. All that we have said about the origin of sensations suggests that the pre-existing mental image is a figment of the psychologist's imagination, just as a pre-existing pain when I suffer from a toothache. Neither the tooth, nor the brain, nor even the mind, contains a series of twinges of pain waiting to be called up. When the appropriate stimulus affects the nerve the pain is the mental indication of the awakened impulses. If I get an image of the dentist, or retrospectively imagine the pain after the tooth is extracted, this is because the necessary conditions have been awakened. There is no more reason to suppose the pre-existing image of the dentist than a pre-existing system of twinges. To assume that images are stored in the brain, is about as reasonable as to assume that flowers and fruit are enclosed in an apple seed, since under suitable conditions these will subsequently arise when the seed is planted. Again, philosophers sometimes assert that the present is big with the future, but not even a philosopher supposes that future events are really existent in the present. What is meant when we think of events as being in the womb of time is that a set of conditions now present will, when combined with future conditions, account for the future event. Similarly when a psychologist thinks of an image as being ' stored up ' all he ought to mean, if he means anything at all, is that the present state of mind together with some future condition will yield the consciousness of an image.

Perhaps this notion of images in the wings waiting to appear on the stage of consciousness, reaches its greatest absurdity when it is assumed that kinesthetic images are the necessary preliminary to a voluntary movement. It is supposed that when I wish to move my limbs I release a pre-existing image of the movement from the cortex of my brain, which passes into the motor area of the cortex and so stimulates the appropriate movement *via* the motor tracts. A similar sort of thing is more often supposed to happen when I wish to speak. The word images are thought of as stored up in the convolutions of the left temporal lobe of the brain, and are released in order to produce speech. This sounds almost too ludicrous for anybody ever to have held, yet it is the basis of much that is believed by psychologists and physicians about aphasia. We shall consider this matter in detail later on, but the fact that it is necessary to consider it at all is due to the widespread belief in the dogma. If it is palpably absurd to assume that word-images lie dormant in the brain prior to their arousal in speech, why is it considered reasonable to suppose that other images behave in this way?

The upshot of the whole matter may be summarized in the statement of Dr Adrian : " Perhaps some drastic revision of our systems of knowledge will explain how a pattern of nervous impulses can cause a thought. If such a revision is made I can only hope that I may be able to understand it." But this hope is doomed for ever not to be realized, since nobody will ever be able to understand it, for the assumed causal relationship between the two events is due to a mistake. Sensations and images are data. We must, as psychologists, start with some material, and these are part of what we start with. They are given in experience and we cannot psychologically go behind them ; they are for us ultimate. *Ex nihilo nihil fit.* Unless we have sensations and images we cannot, as psychologists, make any progress. Of course we can investigate the conditions under which they arise, and it is the psychologist's business (unless it is the physiologist's) to do so. The most immediate of such conditions, on the physiological side, as far as sensations are concerned, are the nervous impulses we have studied. If we abandon the notion of causal efficacy, and consider the relation between the emergence of a sensation and its conditions, the difficulty does not occur. When an artist proceeds to paint a portrait he must fulfil certain conditions, such as mixing his paints, preparing his canvas, posing the sitter, etc. But none of these is the cause of the likeness. They are merely some of the necessary conditions without which, no matter how skilful the artist, the portrait could not emerge from the paint. A famous artist on being asked how he got his effects replied, " Genius, sir, genius ". I suggest that physiologist can only offer a similar reply when asked to explain how a pattern of impulses of a like kind produces a variety of sensations. What the physiologist investigates is physiology. After we have studied all that physiology can teach us about nervous impulses we are still not a whit nearer the sensation, which is left on our hands unexplained and unaccounted for.

Having now reviewed the nature of the nerve impulse and what it cannot do, it remains to consider what it can do. We owe much of our knowledge in this respect to the Russian physiologist J. P. Pavlov (4) and his collaborators, who have opened up a new and interesting chapter in psychological physiology by their work on the so-called conditioned reflexes. Pavlov is a firm and avowed adherent of Descartes' view, that mental factors play no part in such reflexes, and he asserts emphatically that all physiological action, the highest as well as the lowest, is rigidly determined. All is the mechanical result of the appropriate stimuli and there is no room for psychical interference. Now if it can be shewn that even conditioned reflexes cannot be understood without psychical factors, we may well doubt whether purely physiological explanations of living phenomena are ever possible.

There are certain inborn reflexes, of which a good example is the secretion of saliva when food or a noxious substance, such as acid, is placed in the mouth. In the former case the saliva helps to digest the food, in the latter to wash out the noxious object. Such inborn reflexes are very few in number, depending, as they do, on the chemical and physical properties of the agencies acting on the organism directly. It is evident that an animal, endowed with only inborn reflexes, would not long survive, for their activity is dependent on direct contact of certain stimuli with the receptor organs. In the complex conditions of existence it is essential that the approach of physical or chemical stimuli should be signalled to the animal before they reach him, in order to enable him to cope with the coming situation. As the result of individual experience the smell or the sight of food acquire the property of symbols or signals, to stimulate the salivary reaction before the food is tasted. That such responses to signalling stimuli have to be learnt has been shewn by feeding puppies on milk for a few months, when it was found that the sight or smell of bread or meat produced no salivary secretion. Signalling stimuli have become substitutes for what we may call native stimuli, as the result of the animal's experience. Pavlov maintains " that the fundamental and most general function of the hemispheres is that of reacting to signals presented by innumerable stimuli of interchangeable significance." The brain, that is to say, is an organ for the substitution of dissimilars.

Now the animal must take active notice of the signals. If he behaved as a stock or stone the substitution would not occur. This is not surmise but founded on actual observation. Pavlov and his pupils have studied the conditions necessary for substituting a novel stimulus for the native stimuli. They found that an alert state of the animal was absolutely essential in order to effect the substitution. If the animal is drowsy, or irritated, or in a bad state of health, it is difficult, if not impossible, to substitute one stimulus for another. So that at the very outset a psychica lfactor, namely *attention*, plays an essential part in the process. It is very easy to ignore this factor since it is always present, just as a physiological explanation of vision devoted entirely to the structure of the eye and the optic nerves would omit to state that sufficient light to see by is an indispensable factor for seeing things. Attention, of a greater or less degree, is present in every event that can be called mental. What is present in all cases is easily overlooked, and physiologists can hardly be expected to remember what psychologists so persistently forget, that attention is the very kernel of mental happenings.

A very delicate quantitative method has been devised for

studying the effect of a stimulus in producing a conditioned reflex action. The salivary duct of an animal is transplanted from the mouth to the outside of the jaw, or neck, by an incision in the skin. To the opening of the duct there is adjusted a small glass bulb connected to a graduated tube, by means of which the volume of saliva may be accurately measured. In order to avoid the chance of the animal's attention being diverted by extraneous stimuli the work is carried on in sound proof rooms ; the animal and the experimenter being in different compartments. In this manner the effect of various signalling or substitution stimuli may be studied. As the formation and maintenance of acquired reflexes is subject to a number of definite conditions such reflexes are called conditioned reflexes.

It is here necessary to call attention to an ambiguity in the meaning of the term ' stimulus ', the neglect of which leads to much confusion between the physiological and psychological standpoints. For physiological purposes a stimulus has been defined as " any change in the environment of an excitable tissue which, if sufficiently intense, will excite the tissue ". This is a sound scientific definition and indicates exactly what the physiologist does when he stimulates a nerve. As to the relation between a physiological stimulus and the response thereto, except for the ' all or none ' rule we are very much in the dark. For, as Dr Haldane (5) has pointed out, " when we attempt to trace a connection we are lost in an indefinite maze of complex conditions, out of which the response emerges. It is of little use to point out that in many cases the determining cause of a physical change may be something very small as compared with its effect. The turning of a switch or opening of a valve, or the application of a tiny spark, may, for instance, produce gigantic effects. In all these cases we can trace the chain of cause and effect, whereas in the physiological case we cannot. Let it be granted that hope may be entertained of some day tracing the physiological chain. It is nevertheless clear that the existence of such a hope, however confidently expressed, must not be confused with evidence."

Yet the psychologist has adopted the term stimulus and

works it to death. For him it may mean almost anything ; and this extension of its scope robs it of any significance. Thus, if a man responds to the smell of food by secreting saliva the smell is rightly called the stimulus. But if he responds to a threatened blow by running away, or hitting out, the whole situation, or some particular part of it, is also called the stimulus. When he reacts in a theatre by applause, or to a letter by writing a reply, both the play and the letter are called stimuli. What possible utility, for explanatory purposes, can there be in a term of such indefinite significance ? The matter becomes worse when a similarity is assumed between physiological and psychological responses, and deductions are drawn for which the sole justification is the ambiguity of terminology. Human beings, and all animals endowed with a nervous system, respond to total situations or to the meaning of a state of affairs. There are occasions, of course, when they can be accurately said to respond to stimuli in the physiological sense of the term. Amongst these are the responses of the lower senses, such as smell or taste. To these a man responds by physiological reactions, such as sniffing, or secreting saliva. In a similar manner he may react, by a reflex action, to any sudden or violent change, such as an intense noise, or a flash of light, or a burn. Normally, however, the response is made to the acquired meaning of a situation expressed or implied. This will explain a man's totally different response to a bear at large and to a bear in a modern zoological garden. As has been wittily said, to the one he presents a bun, to the other a clean pair of heels. The bear, quâ stimulus, is the same appearance in both cases, but the meaning of the appearance is totally different ; and it is to the meaning of the situation that the man reacts. To call both, objects and the meaning of situations, by the same term leads to such confusion that it would seem desirable, if it were possible, to drop the word stimulus from psychological discussions. Most of the stimuli which the external world rains down on a man are completely ignored by him. His mental life consists in selecting amongst the implied meanings those which will serve his purposes. The motive, in other words, precedes the so-called stimulus which cannot therefore be a cause of it. On the few occasions when the term can be rigidly applied to human activity we are dealing with physiological matters in which the psychological interest is reduced to a minimum.

The notion of a stimulus as causing a response serves to emphasize the fundamental opposition between the physiological and the psychological standpoints. In the former the stimulus is rightly regarded as the cause or determining factor of the ensuing activity, but the real cause of psychological action is the individual acting. Since conduct originates in the organism, in its impulses and desires, it is a psychological blunder to make any use of the term stimulus in the physiological sense when considering human motivation. This has been put very pithily by Professor L. L. Thurstone (6) who says : " I suggest that we dethrone the stimulus. He is only nominally the ruler in psychology. The real ruler of the domain which psychology studies is the individual and his motives, desires, wants, ambitions, cravings, aspirations. The stimulus is merely the more or less accidental fact in the environment, and it becomes a stimulus only when it serves as a tool for somebody's purposes. It is not a cause. It is simply a means by which we achieve our own ends, not those of the stimulus." He illustrates this by considering the rôle of the so-called stimulus in instinctive acts, and concludes that the stimulus cannot be the cause of such acts, but simply a factor which modifies them. He does not go so far as to suggest, as I have done, that the use of the term should be discontinued, but he gives such an appropriate illustration that I quote it. " If you have been walking in the country for hours without companionship, it is not unnatural to find yourself interested in the first stranger you meet. In your customary environment you may have limited your companionship to those of your own kind, ignoring those who differ from you markedly. To say that the stranger is a stimulus to whom you respond as a reactor is to lose the psychologically most important aspect of the situation, namely, your impulse and readiness to be social."

It is time to consider what conditions must be fulfilled in order that a conditioned reflex may arise. The general method of procedure, in substituting one stimulus for another, is quite straightforward. A signalling stimulus, such as an electric shock, the sound of a bell, a metronome beat or a coloured disc, or any other random thing is presented, and immediately afterwards the animal is given food. If this procedure is repeated often enough the animal responds to the signalling stimulus by secreting saliva, even in the absence of food ; and the amount of such secretion is measured in the manner stated above This reaction to the signalling stimulus is called the conditioned reflex, whereas the reaction to the native stimulus is the unconditioned reflex. Conditioned reflexes have been studied in man by fixing a suction disc attached to a tube over the duct of the salivary gland and measuring the number of drops of saliva produced in response to various signalling stimuli. Or, by resting the man's foot on an electrode, it has been found that, if we combine the electric shock with some innocuous stimulus, such as the sound of a bell, sufficiently often, the sound alone will ultimately produce the jerking away of the foot. It has been found possible in this way to determine the limits of infra-red and ultra-violet vision by combining these stimuli with electric shocks and noting the responses.

A little reflection will shew that this is one of the methods by which a child learns to interpret his physical environment. Thus the notion of solidity or resistance of objects originally rests on tactile and muscular stimuli, but, as the result of repeated experiences, visual stimuli of light and shade become adequate signals to arouse the idea of solidity when the object is not near enough to be touched. The visual stimulus acts as a conditioned stimulus for the original unconditioned touch and movement. In a similar fashion Berkeley has shewn that our conditioned perception of distance, or depth, by vision, rests on unconditioned tactual and motor experiences. Motor stimuli are necessary for the original perception of distance, but as a result of their constant union with visual stimuli it comes about that the latter alone act as signals to produce the perception of distance. Childish fears are usually developed in a very similar way. It has been demonstrated that normal children, below the age of one year, have no fear of animals, but they have an innate fear of loud noises. If, then, a barking dog approaches a child suddenly it may happen that on future occasions the mere sight of the dog is sufficient to arouse the emotion of fear. Again, in learning to speak and to understand single words the process is very similar. Words are connected by frequent repetition with internal and external stimuli of every kind. When the union is made, speech comes to serve as a signal for all these, and can alone call forth all the reactions which are natively brought about by the objects themselves. Words are the substitutes for physical or mental objects. Learning by experience is thus, in the main, the ability to substitute one set of stimuli for another, or getting to know the signals for appropriate action. But it should be carefully noted that this only applies to learning at the perceptual level.

The conditions for establishing substituted stimuli have been very carefully studied by Pavlov. He has demonstrated, experimentally, that any stimulus which is to become a signal for a conditioned reflex must begin to operate before the unconditioned stimulus comes into action, and must overlap it in time. For example, the rotation of a circle in front of a dog *before* feeding him produced the salivary reflex after five repetitions only, whilst the sound of an electric bell set going five seconds *after* feeding failed to establish the reflex with four hundred trials. It appears then that the unconditioned stimulus in some way or other inhibits the action of the conditioned. The second condition for establishing conditioned reflexes has already been mentioned, namely, an alert state of the animal, without distraction.

Now let us enquire as to the significance of these two conditions and their implications. Psychologists distinguish between passive or non-volitional attention and active or volitional attention. In the former case we attend willy-nilly and the attention is, as it were, wrung out of us. When a man is thirsty he must notice it whether he wants to or not ; it

obtrudes itself, as we say, on his attention. The attention
he gives to the means necessary to slake his thirst is, however,
of the voluntary kind. It is obvious that any unconditioned
stimulus must by the nature of the case attract non-volitional
attention, since it is always connected with a vital need of
the organism. A signalling stimulus, on the other hand,
unless it is very intense or obtrusive can only secure voluntary
attention, not the passive variety. That is to say, an unconditioned stimulus secures attention by its own nature ; a
conditioned stimulus by its vigour or by its acquired significance. When a hungry animal receives food his whole
attention is absorbed by it and he has none to spare for neutral
or conditioned stimuli. In order to secure attention for a
conditioned stimulus it must have the field to itself, if it is to
come into the animal's focus of consciousness at all. When
this happens, and food is subsequently given whilst the
conditioned stimulus is all the while acting, both the signal
and the food become part of the same attention-process.
If, however, the food is given first, the conditioned stimulus
would not be attended to. It has also been pointed out, above,
that the animal must be in a suitably alert frame of mind.
We see then that the two essential conditions for producing
a conditioned reflex are also the necessary conditions for
securing the animal's attention to the combined stimuli.
The necessity of a fixed order of presentation of the two
stimuli can thus be reasonably explained on psychological
grounds, whereas on purely physiological grounds the order
of events necessary to establish a conditioned reflex seems
entirely arbitrary, not to say miraculous.

Just as a terrible sight may stop the heart, pale the skin,
and cause the hair to stand on end, so the subsequent thought
of the same situation may produce similar physiological
effects. In the same way the mere image of sucking a lemon
will produce a flow of saliva almost as copious as the actual
lemon itself. Now suppose that a signalling stimulus and an
unconditioned stimulus, in that order, have formed part of
the same attention-process on several occasions. We may say
that the animal has attended to a certain configuration of

stimuli. By the law of association, when, on a subsequent
occasion, one part of the configuration is presented the whole
configuration will tend to reinstate itself. If a red disc is
placed before a dog for some time, and he is then fed whilst
the disc is still in his view, the configuration is red disc, food,
flow of saliva. After several trials the red disc alone may be
exhibited and, by virtue of the law of association, food is
anticipated and the saliva begins to flow. Thus the conditioned
reflex is but another name for the psychological law of association. The assimilation of the conditioned reflex to the law
of association is well shewn by the following observation.
When morphine is injected into an animal, it produces nausea,
vomiting and a profuse flow of saliva, followed by sleep.
If the operation is repeated for several days, then the mere
sight of the preparation of the syringe, or even the bare
appearance of the operator, will produce all the symptoms.
The sight of the operator is one of the factors of a total
configuration which, by itself, is adequate to reproduce the
whole original state of affairs. Wise physicians often inject
water into patients instead of morphia in order to produce
sleep. Perhaps it will be objected to the above explanation
that the law of association is entirely a neural law and that
we can dispense with psychical factors. Since, however, this
law was known long before so-called ' association fibres ' were
dreamt of, it is beyond belief that psychologists should have
anticipated brain anatomy solely by psychological introspection and reflection. In any case, the law of association
is unintelligible without the factor of attention, and nobody
has yet discovered a physiological basis for this.

It is instructive to observe that Mr E. R. Guthrie (7) on
independent grounds has come to the same conclusion as
mine, namely that the conditioned reflex is another name for
' association by contiguity in time.' The only objection I have
to this view is that there can be no association of this kind ;
but that all association is due to continuity of interest or
attention. He believes that all the laws of learning can be
reduced to the one formula of association ; or as he says
that the facts of learning may all be cited as examples of

conditioning. He appears to think, however, that the law of association is entirely explicable in terms of brain physiology, *i.e.* association tracts. But this is a blunder ; as all association depends ultimately on psychical factors. What is not attended to together cannot be associated. Amongst the hosts of stimuli which rain down on us simultaneously we actively select some, and these alone are associated.

A stimulus, or a situation, can produce an action of a reflex nature, but it can equally well produce inhibition. It must be strongly insisted upon that inhibition is just as naturally the result of a stimulus as any other effect. Thus suppose a conditioned salivary reflex is being established ; and, whilst the conditioned stimulus is acting, an extraneous sound or odour or light penetrates the room. There is immediately a weakening or a cessation of the reflex activity. The same inhibitory effect is, of course, brought about if a stranger enters the room, which renders it often impossible to demonstrate the conditioned response by an experimenter to another person. Pavlov explains this by saying that " the animal fixes all its appropriate receptor organs upon the source of disturbance, fastening its gaze upon the disturbing agency and sniffing the air." This is an admirable description of the outward and visible signs of the animal's concentrated attention ; and it is not surprising that he ceases to attend to the experimental stimulus. The above kind of inhibition is called external inhibition to distinguish it from direct inhibition where the conditioned stimulus itself becomes inhibitory. During the process of establishing a conditioned reflex we saw that it was essential for the signalling stimulus to be followed by the unconditioned stimulus. This is called reinforcing the former. After the reflex has been established, it is necessary to reinforce it, from time to time, in order to maintain it in an active state. If, however, the signalling stimulus is repeatedly applied, without reinforcement, there is a progressive weakening and finally complete inhibition of the conditioned reflex. Another method of bringing about inhibition is to combine the conditioned stimulus with a totally new stimulus, when the combination of the two inhibits the reflex although the conditioned stimulus, by itself, is still effective. For example, suppose a salivary reflex is formed in response to a metronome beat. If now a coloured disc is presented a few seconds before the metronome is started, the combination of the two inhibits the salivary flow, although the response can still be obtained to the metronome alone. It is perfectly clear, therefore, that the inhibition of a reflex may be just as naturally the effect of a stimulus as the reflex action itself.

The fundamental importance of inhibition to the welfare of the organism may be realized when it is remembered that inhibition is the very kernel of the process of learning. Without it the reactions of an animal to external stimuli would be crude and not adapted to variations in the environment. Such undifferentiated reactions could hardly enable an animal to survive in any but the simplest surroundings. We may illustrate the necessity of the process of inhibition to learning by giving actual instances of what has been found by experiment. If, for example, a tone of a definite number of vibrations per second is used as a signalling stimulus for a salivary reflex, it is found that many tones, in the neighbourhood of this number of vibrations, acquire the same property and the animal secretes saliva in response to them. The response, therefore, is not sharply differentiated with respect to the stimulus ; for the number of vibrations per second may vary within certain wide limits and yet the reaction will follow. If, however, the original tone is constantly reinforced, *i.e.* always followed by food, whilst the neighbouring tones are never reinforced, the animal soon learns to inhibit the reaction except with regard to the one tone. By this means it has been found possible for a dog to differentiate a tone of 800 vibrations per second from one of 812 vibrations ; he reacted to the one but not to the other. In the same way a conditioned reflex was established to a disc rotating clockwise but the animal reacted, at first, also to one rotating anticlockwise ; but by reinforcing only the former stimulus the response to the latter was inhibited. Similarly the reaction to various geometrical forms is at first crude and undifferentiated ; both a circle and a square producing the same reflex response. But an animal soon learns to distinguish between them, if the necessary condition of reinforcement is employed during the period of training. By graduated steps, a dog who had acquired a conditioned salivary reflex to a circle was able, finally, to distinguish this from an ellipse of equal area and luminosity with the axes in the ratio of 8 to 9. He secreted saliva in response to the circle but inhibited the flow when the ellipse was presented. It has been shewn that in the ability to distinguish shades of luminosity a dog's eye is superior to a man's, as it can be taught to discriminate between shades of grey which are quite indistinguishable to the human eye.

The discrimination of shapes, sounds, luminosities, motions, etc., in fact all the variegated array of stimuli which the external world offers to the senses, depends on the power of inhibition. Without it learning would be impossible ; for all sights would lead to similar reactions, all sounds to the same responses and all motions would call forth the same activities from the organism. As we descend in the scale of living things we observe that the excitatory effects of stimuli are much more diffuse, producing irradiating effects over a wide area of the body. Amongst the higher animals such diffuse unco-ordinated action is replaced by activity restricted to definite organs. Within such circumscribed areas of response every individual learns, by his own experience, to respond to finer grades of stimulation by suppressing superfluous reactions. We may presume that the physiological basis of such discrimination is the formation, within the sense organs and nervous system, of series of isochronous fibres whereby the nervous impulses are restricted to definite neurons. The rest of the fibres, falling outside this limited series, have different chronaxies and so do not have the same resonance. Inhibition is thus a fundamental vital process by means of which the nervous system is gradually attuned to the harmonies of the environment. Without the elimination of unnecessary responses by suppression our reactions would fail to be sympathetically attuned to gradations of the stimuli.

In the light of these facts it is preposterous to suppose that there is any psychological ground for the belief that inhibition or suppression can be detrimental to the organism. Yet the psycho-analysts think that all the ills that the mind suffers from originate in suppression. They regard it as a morbid process of an artificial nature and oppose it to the natural process of expression. Hysteria, anxiety-neuroses, obsessions and other nervous illnesses are said to be all due to suppression and can be cured by dragging up the suppressed material. But we have shown that both expression and suppression are equally fundamental. It would, indeed, be paradoxical if a process which lies at the root of all our learning by experience could be harmful. No doubt learning is a tiresome process but it cannot be presumed to be injurious. If, then, there is any reason to believe that suppression may cause nervous disease the grounds for this belief must be other than psychological.

Inhibition may be regarded as a partial sleep, and full sleep is widely irradiated internal inhibition. It was mentioned above that if a conditioned stimulus was repeatedly applied, without being occasionally reinforced, the conditioned reflex would be inhibited and finally extinguished. The repeated extinction of a reflex in this manner leads to drowsiness. So powerful is this effect that even electric shocks which have acquired conditioned properties have been found, after being repeated for many months without reinforcement, to produce inhibition and finally to induce sleep. We also saw that another method of producing inhibition was to combine a neutral stimulus with a conditioned stimulus. In one experimental case a dog had acquired a salivary reflex in response to the sound of a whistle. During the course of the investigation the sound of bubbling water was occasionally introduced in conjunction with the whistle. As usual the animal was at first alert towards the direction of the new sound, but as the result of frequent repetitions of the combined stimuli he finally became drowsy and fell asleep. It may be objected that inhibition and sleep are mere passive effects and should not be confused with active processes. But this is a mistake,

D

for Pavlov (8) has shewn that sleep involves the controlling activity of the cerebral cortex. He says : " Experiments in our laboratory shewed that while in a normal dog an investigatory reflex (*i.e.* alertness shewn by orienting the body and sense organs) to a definite sound quickly vanished, the same sound in a dog with extirpated cortex, under identical conditions, called forth an investigatory reflex in a stereotyped manner and for an unlimited number of times." Thus inhibition is an active process involving the use of the cortex ; and sleep, or widely irradiated inhibition, demands the co-operation of the higher levels of the nervous system. If, therefore, inhibition or suppression is the real cause of nervous disease no more dangerous occupation could be undertaken than regular nocturnal sleep.

Before leaving the subject of conditioned reflexes it is desirable to call attention to certain facts which seem to me to render invalid any attempt to explain them on mechanical principles. We saw above that, despite all beliefs to the contrary, mental factors are essential to the formation of such reflexes, and we shall return to this topic in a later chapter. Now any mechanical principles would operate uniformly in all animals, just as they do in all machines. But animals do not behave in this way ; each exhibits a certain individuality making his responses different from others. It is only by ignoring these essential variations and by regarding the experiments abstractly that the mechanical explanation can be defended. But Pavlov (9) has demonstrated that, in response to the same stimulus, different animals react differently. They exhibit temperamental variations. Some show excessive tendencies to excitability and others to inhibition, and it is impossible to say, before trial, what will happen to any individual. The transformation of an inhibitory stimulus, for example, into an excitatory one may produce such profound effects that the animal may cease to respond at all even to strong stimuli and even pass into sleep. Only by ignoring these temperamental differences between animals and treating them all as equivalent or interchangeable units can the mechanical view of the nature of conditioned reflexes be rendered at all tolerable as a theory.

The early English economists invented the ' economic man ', a creature who acted solely from utilitarian economic motives. From the assumed simple characteristics of such a being they deduced rigid mechanical economic laws. No matter that people did not behave in accordance with these laws and neither bought in the cheapest market nor sold in the dearest. They were assumed to act in these ways and all their real ways of acting were ignored or tortured into ways which fitted these so-called laws of economic activity. Exactly the same state of affairs prevails in physiology. Animals must behave in accordance with these rigid rules ; and so all temperamental variations are slurred over or denied, and a ' physiological animal ' is substituted for the real animals that live and move and run about and refuse to show pure reflex activities. A physiological dog is one whose actions are completely determinate ; whereas a real dog is a trouble-some creature who very unkindly refuses to play the game.

We have now examined the main postulates of psychological physiology. But it must always be borne in mind that the physiologist deals with bodily functions in an abstract manner, since he isolates them and studies them separately. Vital activity is, however, essentially co-ordinated and integrated activity. It is not to isolated stimuli that the normal animal responds but to complex situations. The reactions of isolated nerves to electrical stimuli, though they help us to analyse the nervous impulse, teach us very little about psychological action. Experiments on conditioned reflexes, since they are performed on the complete animal, are much more instructive ; but they, too, are abstract, since the animal normally responds to the meaning of a total situation and not to artificially isolated stimuli.

CHAPTER III

PHYSIOLOGICAL PSYCHOLOGY—ANIMAL

WE have now passed in review such of the tenets of nerve physiology as are supposed to be essential to the explanation of mental functioning. It is now time to consider the effect on mental functions of injury or disease of the nervous system. In this way it may be possible to put the assumptions to the test of experimental proof. Much of the physiology used by psychology is, as we have suggested, hypothetical and speculative, and invented for specific purposes. For this reason it will be necessary to adhere rigidly to actual experimental data.

It was previously stated that Descartes' views about nervous activity for long held sway. But, as far as English-speaking countries are concerned, the detailed speculations of Hartley (1705–1759) on nerve functioning were unhesitatingly accepted by psychologists all through the nineteenth century and are still widely, if implicitly, held. These views were set out in his *Observations on Man* published in 1749. Hartley (1) took the doctrine of association which was then under discussion by philosophers, and, grafting on to it his own theories about nervous processes, formulated the law of association. With astonishing acumen he invented, out of his own head, a theory of nervous activity which bears a close resemblance to modern views.

Sensations were, for him, the mental equivalent of vibrations in the minute particles of the nervous substance. External objects, by producing light waves or sound waves or other vibrations, communicated these through the sense organs to the nerves, whence they were transferred along the spinal cord to the brain. Images and ideas arose in a similar way, being the equivalent of smaller vibrations. Thus, he said,

" Sensations by being oft repeated, leave certain vestiges, types or images of themselves ", and so sensory vibrations produce in the brain substance " a disposition to diminutive vibrations corresponding to themselves." Hartley was acute enough to see that such vibrations were of a purely mechanical nature, whereas sensations and images are mental ; and he, therefore, affirmed that it was impossible for him to discover in what way the former " cause or are connected with " the latter. It is a great pity that his successors, who owe their nerve physiology to him, did not exercise equal caution. Vesalius, indeed, an anatomist of the sixteenth century, had stated : " How the brain performs its functions in imagination, in reasoning, in thinking and in memory (or in whatever way, following the dogmas of this or that man, you prefer to classify or name the several actions of the chief soul) I can form no opinion whatever. Nor do I think that anything more will be found out by anatomy." (2) Vesalius' prediction has, so far, been verified.

Hartley made a consistent and exhaustive attempt to explain the whole of mental life by the help of his doctrine of sensations and images coupled with the principle of association. His views rapidly spread and were ultimately adopted in their entirety, as regards nervous functioning, by psychologists owing to the influence, first, of the English associationists, and then of William James. (3) The latter took them over completely and explained association in terms of brain processes, thus : " When two elementary brain processes have been active together or in immediate succession, one of them, on re-occurring, tends to propagate its excitement into the other." In a similar fashion it is easy to account for memory, since it was assumed that retention and recollection are simply the stamping in of impressions in the brain and their subsequent arousal by some association path. The phenomena of habit and instinct were, and are, still explained by the doctrine of neural pathways or patterns. Imagination is a little more difficult, but if Hartley's view is adopted that images are only faint sensations there is no insuperable obstacle to a neural explanation. Thus James stated : " All we need suppose is that intra-cortical currents are unable to produce in the cells the strong explosions which currents from the sense organs occasion, to account for the subjective differences between images and sensations, without supposing any difference in their local seats. To the strong degree of explosion corresponds the character of ' vividness ' or sensible presence, in the subject of thought ; to the weak degree, that of ' faintness ' or outward unreality." This belief is still the accepted foundation of the explanation of the origin of images by psychological physiology.

It is evident that the above explanations rest upon the assumption we have already dealt with, namely that there must be a point-to-point correspondence between brain states and mental events, and also that any quantitative characteristics of the one must be reflected in the other. But images as we have insisted are different in kind from sensations and are not merely different in intensity, since it is possible to have an image of a sensation of minimal intensity. And we have seen that by the ' all or none ' rule the strength of the nervous impulse is not dependent on the intensity of the stimulus. All that a stronger ' explosion ' could do would be to bring more fibres into play, so that we should be reduced to the absurdity of supposing that the difference between an image and a sensation was due to the number of nervous fibres involved in their production. Underlying the whole of this conception of the relation between mental and nervous events there is the implied dogma that the former is in some way or other a photographic reproduction of the latter.

The notion of fixed ' pathways ' or ' traces ' in the nervous system to account for memory, habit, instinct, etc., is still widely held. The ' pathways ' are nowadays usually conceived as constituted by fixed reflex ' patterns ', but the underlying conception is exactly the same. Thus Professor J. B. Watson (4) says : " Instinct and habit are undoubtedly composed of the same elementary reflexes. They differ so far as concerns the origin of the pattern and order of unfolding of the elements composing the pattern. In instinct the pattern and order are inherited, in habit both are acquired during the life-time of the individual. We can define habit then as we did instinct as a complex system of reflexes which functions in a serial order." This whole explanation rests upon the tacit assumption that habit and instinct are fixed responses to unvarying situations. But both habit and instinct are infinitely plastic, adapting themselves to varying situations ; as the same situations rarely, if ever, occur. In any habitual reaction the response is, at once, adapted to changes in the perceived situation, and the same is true of instinct. (5) The important thing to be emphasized is that the physiology underlying all such explanations is almost entirely speculative. The observed facts are facts of behaviour and the physiology is invented in order to supply a physical basis, without which no explanation is considered adequate or scientific.

We shall now consider whether there is any experimental evidence to justify the theory that there are definite patterns or fixed pathways in the central nervous system. The experiments have, for the most part, been conducted on lower animals, such as rodents, and it is naturally hazardous to make inferences from these to man. If, however, the theory of evolution is true, we must believe that the complicated brain of a human being has developed out of a similar type of nervous system, and comparative anatomy and embryology shews this to be correct. We have also seen that the physiologist supposes that in the higher animals no essentially new functions of the brain arise, but that the complications which ensue are the elementary functions of conveying impulses raised, as it were, to a higher power. It is reasonable, therefore, to assume that the capacities exhibited by the nervous system of the lower animals are still present as possibilities in the human brain. That is to say, if it can be shown, for instance, that various parts of the brain are functionally interchangeable in the lower animals the probability is that the human brain possesses the same latent power.

The functions of the brain are best studied by cultivating a habit in some animal and determining the conditions under which it is lost or retained. A straightforward way of doing this is to place the animal in a simple ' maze ' consisting of a central compartment out of which there are alternative paths, one leading to a cul-de-sac and the other to a dish of food. A hungry animal finding itself in such a maze, sooner or later learns to go straight to the food without entering the blind alley. A record is kept of the time taken to reach the food and the number of errors, *i.e.* the number of times he selects the wrong path. The animal is regarded as having acquired the habit when, on several successive trials, say ten, he gets the food without making an error. It must be remembered, too, that an essential feature in acquiring a habit is the elimination of fumbling and unnecessary movements, as is seen, for instance, in the gracefulness and ease of an accomplished dancer when compared with the awkward sprawling of a tyro.

Messrs S. I. Franz and K. S. Lashley (6) trained a number of white rats in such a simple maze as we have described until they could traverse the path and get the food without making a mistake. Some of the animals were overtrained, that is they had a considerable amount of practice after they had learnt the task completely. When the training had been successfully accomplished the frontal portion of the brain was excised under ether, as it is probable that, in these animals, the ' motor area ' is situated in that region. The extent of the lesion was, in all cases, determined by a post-mortem microscopical examination. After the operation the animals were again tested. A comparison was then made of the time taken and the number of errors in the first fifteen trials after the operation, and the first fifteen trials during the original learning period. It was found that the trained animals required about a third less time and made about half as many mistakes after the destruction of the frontal lobes, whilst the overtrained animals took ninety per cent. less time and made ninety per cent. fewer errors. The loss in capacity, which in the overtrained group is practically negligible, is probably due to the shock effects of the operation. It is noteworthy that none of the animals exhibited the exploratory sniffings at corners and cracks and the fumbling which is so characteristic of untrained rats. However we explain the slight loss, it is evident that there is a considerable amount of retention of the habit. After a fortnight the animals were again subjected to a second operation, in which the dorsal and lateral regions of the cortex were excised, leaving only the occipital portion. Yet there was considerable retention of the habit although only about one-third of the cortex remained. (7)

When we pass to more complicated habits a different conclusion is reached. Some of the animals, whose frontal lobes were completely or partially destroyed, were trained to get food from a box by climbing to the top, depressing a plane which opened the door, and then climbing down again to the door. Complete destruction of the frontal lobes resulted in the loss of the habit ; but the habit was retained when other parts of the brain were destroyed, or when some portion only of the frontal lobe was intact. The experimenters concluded that " although some part of the frontal region must remain intact if the plane-box habit acquired by normal animals is to be retained, the particular part preserved is immaterial. The different parts of the frontal region are . . . equipotential in the functioning of the habit." These investigations go far to overthrow any belief in a strict localization of function in the cortex and consequently tend to invalidate the belief in the theory of ' centres ' subserving such mental functions. For, after destruction of all parts of the cortex to which the function of habit-formation has been assigned, such as the frontal, temporal, parietal or orbital, it was found that the albino rat still retains and can form simple habits. Hence the conclusion seems justified that " the ability of the animals to form habits after the loss of those parts of the brain which are normally used in learning, the re-establishment of motor control after the loss of the stimulable area of the cortex and of the corpus striatum, and the seeming equipotentiality of the different parts of the frontal pole in the functioning of complex habits go far towards establishing the complete functional interchangeability of all parts of the cerebral cortex." If this deduction is too rash, at all events it rests on experimental evidence, whereas the contrary view is entirely a matter of speculation.

Experiments similar to those we have described have been further elaborated by K. S. Lashley, and as they deal with still more complicated habits they will be next considered. He took a number of rats, in groups, and destroyed a definite area of the cortex in each group; varying the position, so that all regions of the cortex were destroyed in one or other of the groups. Thus, in some group one hemisphere was removed, in another both occipital regions, in a third both parietal regions, or both parietal and frontal areas, and so forth. The extent of the injury was determined in all cases by a subsequent post-mortem microscopical examination. The animals were trained to open a box enclosed in a cage, which could only be done by depressing in a fixed order two latches attached to platforms at opposite ends of the box. If the order was reversed the box could not be opened. The number of trials required by each animal to perform the trick successfully, without any error, was observed, and compared with the number required by a control group of normal uninjured rats. The astonishing result was found that, whilst the normal animals required, on the average, about 140 trials the average number for the operated animals was about 80. In nearly all cases the animals with the maximum lesion learnt the habit more quickly than the others. This paradoxical result apparently proves too much, until we remember that one part of the brain may exercise an inhibitory influence over the rest. Lashley, however, thinks that the result is a chance one due to the fact that the uninjured animals were much more vigorous than the others and when they reached the platforms they tended to jump over them instead of depressing the latches, whilst the operated animals do not do this. Subsequent experiments with different animals have shewn that the rate of formation of this habit is not influenced by any cortical injury up to fifty per cent., and is independent of the locus of the lesion. Both normal and operated animals learn at the same rate.

An important quantitative result has been reached in

experiments with a maze of a more complicated form than that above mentioned. (8) The maze had eight culs-de-sac requiring alternate right and left turns in order to reach the food. Twenty-one rats were operated upon and the extent of the cerebral lesion was subsequently carefully determined in each case. The total surface area of the cerebrum excised in different animals, in various regions, ranged from one and a half to eighty-one per cent., and the animals were given five trials a day until ten consecutive errorless trials were obtained. Estimates of the amount of practice required for complete learning were made by taking into account the total time taken in all the trials, the number of errors, and the number of trials. Statistical correlations were then computed between the amount of practice and the magnitude of the injury. The correspondence was so close that it was inferred that the ability to learn a complicated habit of this kind is a direct function of the quantity of cerebral tissue uninjured. The retardation in learning seems to depend, therefore, on the extent of the destruction, irrespective of its locus within the cerebral hemispheres. So that we are led again to the view that the functions of different cerebral areas are qualitatively the same.

It has sometimes been thought that when a habit is formed the movements, which were previously controlled by the cortex, are taken over by the deep-lying structures. But this view is negatived by the fact that in the different experiments extensive destruction of such structures took place. " In the various tests practically every deep-lying structure above the thalamus was injured and it seems clear that none of these cerebral nuclei is of greater importance for learning than is the pallium."

Great caution should be exercised in interpreting such investigations as these. We may safely conclude, however, that whatever else the numerical results shew they, at least, demonstrate that the injured animals are still able to learn a complicated habit though it may be less readily than the uninjured. Moreover, extensive destruction of the cortex, amounting to four-fifths in some cases, only entails a correlated slowness in the animal's learning capacity. The capacity to acquire the maze habit, for instance, is dependent on the amount of cortical tissue and not upon its anatomical specialization.

Partially decerebrate animals are therefore not incapable of learning or retaining habits ; and any specific portion of the cerebrum can be dispensed with in acquiring complex activities. Thus the various regions of the cortex seem to be equipotential, as far as experiment can ascertain. This must not necessarily be interpreted to mean that definite portions of the cortex play no specific rôle in our ordinary activities. If my right hand is injured I can learn to write with my left or even with my toes, and armless painters have been known to paint with a brush in their mouths. Normally, as a result of evolution or of habit, in order to accomplish certain actions impulses traverse specific parts of the brain in preference to others. Consequently any injury to such parts is accompanied by a corresponding loss of function. But the rest of the hemispheres retain their original power of transmitting any impulse, and under appropriate conditions, especially when there is no other alternative, there is a restitution of function. It is clear that such recovery will be more difficult the more the animal is removed from primitive conditions, i.e. the higher he is in the animal scale. And we know as a matter of fact that the higher animals have more difficulty and take a longer time to recover any lost function.

There is one function, namely vision, for which in the higher animals the occipital area of the brain has long been held to be essential. Destruction of this area is said to lead to blindness. Experiments have been tried with a discrimination-box which offers a choice of alleys at the end of each of which there is a translucent plate. One of these plates is illuminated, the other is kept dark. The animal secures food if he chooses the bright plate and gets a shock if he goes to the dark alley. After the habit of brightness-discrimination had been established in three groups of animals, the frontal, the parietal and the occipital areas respectively were destroyed. Both the former groups retained the habit after the operation, but the latter group lost it completely. Nevertheless a couple of these animals were found capable of relearning the habit in the normal time. And in a subsequent investigation, a dozen of the animals who had partially lost the complicated maze habit, owing to destruction of various parts of the cerebrum, were subsequently trained in the habit of brightness-discrimination. They proved to be in no way inferior to normal animals in acquiring the latter habit despite a considerable loss of tissue in many cases in the occipital *area striata*. (9) Thus it would appear that vision is possible in rats in the absence of the occipital areas.

With regard to the higher animals the evidence for the connection between the mesial part of the occipital lobe (*area striata*) and vision is most conflicting. (10) It was originally thought that destruction of any part of this area produced a local permanent blindness (cortical blindness) corresponding in position to the locus of injury. Each retinal area was supposed to be represented in a corresponding functional area in the occipital cortex. In fact this assumed connection between the retina and the cortex was largely responsible for the idea of a point-to-point correspondence between the functions of the body and the mind. Later observation and experiment have not confirmed the earlier beliefs. It was found that partial extirpation of both occipital areas in dogs resulted in disturbance of vision which was uniform for the entire area of both retinas, and not localized. Again, any part of the occipital cortex may be destroyed without any loss of vision. E. Hitzig studied over one hundred cases of occipital injury and found no accurate projection of the retina on the cortex, but only a tendency for representation of each quadrant, with much individual variation. The partial blindness sometimes resulting from cortical lesions is rarely permanent, as there is a recovery after a shorter or longer time. Where there appears to be blindness there is often a sensitivity to light, though there may be no perception of objects. M. Minkowski made a careful study of the visual area in the dog and found that the upper and lower halves of the visual field were represented in the lower and upper halves respectively of the *area striata*, but he denied any point-to-point correspondence between the retina and the cortex. He maintains that " every perceptual element of the retina is in relation with a whole area of perceptual elements in the cortex." All that we can say is that there is some sort of representation of the four quadrants of the retina in the cortex. Unless injury to the cortical area involves complete blindness in a quadrant there is recovery of vision. Finally there is reason to believe that similar results to those found in dogs are observable in man. So that even the ' visual area ' of the cortex exhibits equipotentiality of function which we have seen to be a property of other parts of the cerebrum.

We saw in the first chapter that one of the most important assumptions of psychological physiology was this one-to-one correspondence between neural processes and mental events. This assumption has been seized upon by the philosophers and has become a fixed dogma ; and they proceed to erect upon it the most elaborate theories. Such is the way of philosophers who, with unexceptionable logic, discuss the relation of mind to body on the basis of doubtful facts which they accept with dogmatic assurance. In his acute discussion of the applicability of the causal laws to mind Mr W. E. Johnson (11) assumed, as a matter needing no justification whatever, that there was a strict correspondence not only between sensations and their neural accompaniments but also between mental images and their neural processes. He further accepted without question, that the mental process of association was paralleled by an unvarying series of neural correlates, a fixed point-to-point correspondence. He then proceeded, by an ingenious logic, to argue that when a man perceived that two objects are separated in space this is on the basis of neural correlates which correspond spatially to the perception. The spatial relations between the cortical areas stimulated varies " in accordance with some formula " with the spatial relations which the person apprehends. The physiology of the situation stops when the cortical areas are stimulated ; but since the person cognizes the spatial relation, he argued that there can be no neural process corresponding to such cognition. Again when a man compares two objects he may find that they agree or differ or so forth. Now the respects in which the sense experience agree or differ correspond to the respects in which the underlying neural processes agree or differ. But there is no further mode in which the neural processes vary which corresponds to the act of comparison itself. Similar considerations apply to all the higher mental processes. Thus, when a person is thinking by means of language, the association of neural correlates is supposed to account for the association of the words in the sentence. About this we shall have a good deal to say in the next chapter. But, assuming this to be the case, for the sake of argument, Mr Johnson rightly remarks that a sentence is not merely a string of words but a significant whole. And neural associations cannot account for the added mental fact that the sentence is understood as having a meaning. Thus, whilst the *data* of mental events may have neural correlates the higher processes of judgment, reasoning, etc., are all devoid of them.

This reasoning seems to me quite sound although the premisses are invalid. Dr C. D. Broad (12), however, expresses himself as astonished at it and, since he cannot impugn the logic, he proceeds to attack the underlying physiology. What Mr Johnson has maintained is that there is a one-to-one correspondence between the *occurrence* of mental states and the occurrence of neural processes. This exhausts all that the neural correlates could possibly account for ; and so, purely subjective activity, such as attention or judgement, can have no nervous basis. Why cannot another part of the cortex be responsible for such subjective acts as attention or judgement, asks Dr Broad ? Well, we saw in Chapter I that Dr Elliot Smith provided such an organ in the prefrontal area ; but this was because he did not know what else to do with it. It is an astonishing psychology which wants organs for naked activities. What can attention be like if there is nothing to attend to ? Set the organ to work and what is the resulting activity ? Even the faculty psychologists could not do much with a faculty of attention. But Dr Broad is not quite happy about putting these faculties in different cortical areas. So he invents a new sort of physiological action. Just as a metal globe, if sufficiently heated, gives off both heat and light by diverse actions, so a cortical area gives rise both to sensations and to judgements about them. Physiology knows nothing about these diverse activities of the same area, but so much the worse for a science which cannot perform the simple operation of imagining a faculty of judgement *in abstracto*. Stimulate a cortical centre at one degree of intensity and a judgement is evoked. Now stimulate it at a higher degree, in defiance of the all or none rule, and you give it something to judge about. How astonished the astonishment neural correlate must be when it perceives the judgement area merely engaged in judging without any terms to judge about ! Perhaps we had better rely on the physiologists after all to provide us with our psychology rather than on philosophers.

Lashley, to whom we owe much of our exact knowledge on the subject of cortical localization reasonably enough concludes that there is a possibility of complete vicarious functioning in all parts of the cerebrum and the underlying nuclei. Any specialization of function is only relative, and learning can proceed, sometimes with undiminished efficiency, in the absence of such specialized areas. I cannot do better than quote his words. " The possibility," he says, " is not excluded by any evidence that I know of that the loss of motor control in paralysis is due, not to the interruption of conditioned reflex paths, but to some disturbance in tonic innervation [he might have said to some disturbance in the chronaxies of the nerve fibres]. The loss of voluntary movement in hemiplegia, pure motor aphasia, etc., might thus be due solely to the disturbance of some fundamental co-ordinating mechanisms upon which the habitual reactions are superimposed rather than to interruption of the habit-mechanisms themselves." One conclusion emerges unmistakably, namely, that the dogma of a point-to-point correspondence between brain structure and psychological functioning rests on no solid foundation whatever.

Objection may be taken to the conclusions just reached on

the ground that it is hazardous to make any inference from the behaviour of lower animals to man. Such objection can hardly be raised to deductions from observations on monkeys whose nervous systems are sufficiently similar to our own to justify the belief that their functions are similar. In order to determine the best methods of treatment for human paralysis, experiments were carried out on four young male monkeys (*macacus rhesus*). (13) Under ether anæsthesia the extent of the ' motor area ' of the cortex was determined by stimulation, and completely destroyed by electric thermo-cautery ; the destruction extending to the motor zone lying within the central fissure and also beyond the motor area. The left motor cortex was destroyed in the case of one monkey and, of course, complete hemiplegia of the right side of the body ensued. The left arm was bandaged so that it could not be used, whilst the limbs of the right side were agitated by striking and the muscles and nerves stimulated by constant friction. By this procedure the animal was left with no alternative but was forced to try to use his paralysed limbs ; and soon began to do so. In a fortnight he began to use the arm for grasping food and the leg for climbing and holding. After three weeks he could pick up small objects and convey them to his mouth. In about three months he was able to catch a fly with his right hand and his movements were as accurate and forceful as those of a normal monkey. A second similar operation was now performed on the right hemisphere, but this time the left side was given no special treatment nor was the recovered right arm restrained. The left arm remained without much capacity for six months, except that it came into use when the animal was emotionally excited in any way.

Thus, by compelling the animal to use a limb and assisting him by the stimulation of the peripheral muscles and nerves, or by emotional excitement, recovery takes place to such an extent that movements are normal. If such methods are not employed, restitution of function is slow and incomplete. In other words when we force an animal to use his mental resources we enable him to overcome his physical disabilities.

E

This provides a clear instance of the primacy of mental factors in bodily functioning. It may be presumed that in other cases, where permanent loss of function has been observed as the result of brain lesions, the loss is partially due to the fact that no mental stimulus has been given sufficiently powerful to awaken the function.

In the case of the second monkey the left motor cortex was destroyed, but the unparalysed left limbs were in no way restrained. The paralysed limbs were not actively stimulated, though they were continually massaged to assist the circulation. There was no restitution of motor ability after a month of this treatment. At the end of this time the right motor area was cauterized and the right arm bound to the body. Active movements of the left limb were invoked by a strong mechanical stimulation. In another month the monkey could use the left side in a normal manner. He used his legs for walking and jumping with accuracy, and recovery was complete and permanent after five months. The third animal had the same operation on the left side and the left arm was strapped so that, as before, the movements of the paralysed side were necessary for feeding and climbing. No treatment was given, the limbs being simply allowed the chance of recovering spontaneously, but there was no return of motor ability for a month. During the next month the nerves and muscles were stimulated by friction and the animal was urged by special strong stimulation to use his arm and leg. As a result of this strenuous treatment his movements became quite normal. A similar result was obtained with the fourth monkey. Right hemiplegia was brought about by cauterizing the left motor cortex, and the left arm was bandaged to the side. The muscles of the right arm, shoulder and leg were stimulated by friction, as also were the corresponding nerves. Irritating exercises were employed to prompt the animal to make defensive movements. This procedure brought about such rapid recovery that after three weeks it was not possible to notice any difference in motor ability on the two sides of the body.

It is now evident that recovery of motor function does not

occur if the animal is left to his own devices. Stimulation of muscle and nerve of the paralysed limbs is necessary. But, what is more important still, is some strong mental incentive. The animal must be induced to use his limbs, either by the desire for food, or to ward off a threatened injury, or by being emotionally excited in some way. In order to make the mental excitement sufficiently powerful he must be debarred from using his unparalysed limbs. When all alternatives are closed to him and he is forced, especially under the influence of emotion, to feed himself or to climb by using his paralysed limbs, he can do so ; otherwise he remains powerless. These observations should make us cautious in accepting any experimental evidence concerning the functions of various regions of the brain unless we have good reason to believe that the mental stimuli necessary to excite the function have been brought into play. So far from mental factors being unnecessary in order to account for bodily activity, as Pavlov and others suppose, the voluntary mechanism is powerless without them.

One of the most firmly held maxims of neurologists is, as was previously stated, that all cortical activity is of the reflex type. But Messrs Franz and Ogden, who performed the above experiments, are surely justified in saying : " It is reasonable to conclude that not all of the recovered motor ability of the monkeys is of the nature of reflexes of a complicated type, and if we conclude that only a few of the recovered movements are ' voluntary ' it is sufficient to cause us to hesitate to accept the generally accepted view of cortical motor functions." The generally accepted belief referred to here is that all brain activity is purely reflex, the inevitable mechanical result of the appropriate mechanical stimulus. On this view a series of impulses cannot be originated in the brain, which simply reflects the impulses originating in the sense organs. But we have now sufficient evidence to shew that even purely reflex acts can only be accounted for by invoking the aid of mental factors. It is also clear that the doctrine of fixed pathways in the central nervous system subserving habitual acts rests on no solid foundation. For the destruction of the original motor paths seems to make no difference to the ultimate activity of the animal. We are further justified in concluding that ' centres ' for particular actions are equally devoid of experimental support, since the elimination of such centres does not entail the disappearance of the function. Finally all theories about ' traces ' in particular cells or areas of the brain whose stimulation produces memories or images rests on no factual evidence, but are a relic of speculative neurology.

The real point at issue, as K. S. Lashley (14) has pointed out, is whether the cerebrum is a highly specialized organ or merely a mass of nervous tissue comparable in all, save complexity, to the spinal cord. In all cases where it has been stated that the formation of habits is not possible in the complete absence of the cerebrum " this conclusion has been advanced without any serious attempt to train the animals, on the basis of the general impression of stupidity given by them. Without careful training such observations are worthless." Even a decerebrate dog can learn to accommodate the stepping movements of his hind legs to follow the movements of a chair on which his forefeet are placed. And it has been shewn that such a dog can seek food and avoid obstacles and shews a marked improvement from month to month in the ability to care for himself. Only careful and prolonged experiment and training, made suitable to the particular species, can decide what an animal can or cannot learn. In this respect complicated habits must be sharply distinguished from very simple ones. Decerebrate animals undoubtedly lose the vast majority of their learned reactions and it is, naturally, difficult for them to acquire new ones. But when the incentive to learn can be made sufficiently strong and the task sufficiently simple, such animals can acquire new modes of activity. We also saw that the destruction of a large part of the cerebrum does not prevent retention of some habits, and this suggests that there are not any specialized centres for learning in the brain.

It has been known for some time that injury to a definite portion of the cortex on the left side of the brain in human beings leads to aphasia or a loss of the function of speech. Re-education, however, is frequently possible and the patient may recover completely or partially. Speech, of course, depends on the co-operation of an enormous number of acquired habits. The efficacy of the re-education of aphasic persons should be measured by comparing the patient's progress with that of a child learning to speak, and not with the speech of an adult. Regarded from this angle recovery from aphasia, in many cases, is astonishingly rapid and complete, though the injury to the brain is permanent ; and this again suggests that there are not special centres for learning in the cortex. We shall revert to this matter in the next chapter.

It was mentioned previously that a widely accepted postulate was that of ' association fibres ' joining definite centres. When certain functions are suspended, owing to brain lesions, it is assumed that the association paths are broken down. Now in order to carry out a voluntary act, such as grasping a seen object, it is necessary to receive certain sensory impressions and to send out efferent impulses to the muscles. The so-called association fibres merely happen to lie anatomically on the usual path of such impulses. When the usual line is interfered with there may be disturbance of function, but as we have now abundantly seen the disturbance is only temporary. Moreover, Lashley cut across the various association fibres in some animals which had learnt the complicated maze habit with eight culs-de-sac. He found that the habit was retained with no serious diminution of efficiency. (15) It is obvious, therefore, that permanent association paths are a mere supposition. The evidence at our disposal strongly suggests that most parts of the cortical hemispheres can take on the function of other parts. In other words complete vicarious functioning is the law of cerebral activity. This being the case the association paths must, like the brain centres, be given up, and we are bound to assume that the whole cortex is capable of facilitating activities of very diverse nature. But although vicarious functioning is always a possibility it by no means follows that it may in all cases become an actuality, especially with human beings. For in such a complicated activity as speech, for example, dependent as it is on the orderly march of a series of co-ordinated impulses to the vocal organs, and made habitual in early childhood, the difficulty of making any change must be enormous.

In this connection the remarks of Lashley are so pertinent that a long quotation is permissible. "Both sensory and intellectual capacities of the adult man are the results of years of training which have led to the establishment of countless habits having a definite structural basis. Cerebral injury may destroy a great number of these, instead of the few which such an animal as the rat has formed, and the apparent loss of function will, therefore, be greater. Further, the rate of learning in the human adult depends largely on the number and complexity of the habits already organized. When the latter are abolished the entire system must be built up *de novo* before anything like an approach to adult performance is attained. The recent studies of re-education in hemiplegia, aphasia and apraxia shew that the loss from the cerebral lesions is never permanent in man and that an unlimited though slowly acquired vicarious functioning is possible. The difference seems to be one of degree rather than of kind. The rat loses less than higher forms because he has less to lose and he seems to recover more rapidly chiefly because a little improvement brings him relatively nearer the standard of comparison (normality) than does the same improvement in man."

The facts dealt with so far make it evident that most, if not all, of the assumptions enumerated in the first chapter are untenable. There remains, however, the doctrine of reflex activity to be more carefully considered. According to this theory all nervous activity, whether at the spinal level or the cortical level is composed of the same units, namely simple reflexes more or less highly integrated. This is supposed to derive its validity from experiments on animals deprived of a brain and possessing only a spinal cord. In such cases there is a certain uniformity of sequence between the stimulus and the response. For example, in a spinal dog irritation of the skin leads to the scratch reflex. This is interpreted to mean that the impulse set up by the stimulus travels along a definitely fixed conduction path in the spinal cord. But this very definiteness is inconsistent with what we have learnt about nervous events in the cortex, and makes it hopeless to apply the reflex conception to facts of behaviour. The distinguishing feature of behaviour is its plasticity; that is, there are no specific excitants, no fixed central paths and no stereotyped reactions. In the brain there are no definitely fixed conduction paths, and the more we attempt to use the reflex theory to explain behaviour the more hopeless it appears. I always raise my arm to ward off a threatened blow, but the danger is never presented twice in the same way and the response is adapted to variations in the total situation. To call a threatened blow a ' stimulus ' and infer from this that it must stimulate ' the same receptors ' is merely a juggling with words. To call all the muscles which have been brought into play ' the effector organs ' is innocuous, unless it is assumed that the impulses have travelled along a predetermined path when it is palpably erroneous, for a host of other reactions have followed, which vary from case to case, and are left out of account. All these latter, however, are an integral part of the reaction. For I sometimes hit out in response to the blow and sometimes retreat ; and it is preposterous to say that I make the ' same reaction ' to the ' same stimulus '. Nor is the difficulty overcome by speaking of a pattern of stimuli to which the reaction is supposed to be a corresponding pattern.

The fact of the matter is that the reflex theory is due to a passion for simplicity, a desire to have simple units to work with. The separation of receptor organs from effectors is a matter of anatomy but corresponds to nothing in living activity. The organism is a unity and responds to any particular situation as a whole. We may, if we choose, separate out parts of the situation and call these the pattern of stimuli ; and parts of the response and name them the pattern of reaction. But this is a pure abstraction. In reality the sensory apparatus and the motor apparatus together constitute a unitary organ for response. If, then, the reflex arc is an artifact there is little to be gained by attempting to apply it to the activity of the cortex. If I turn my head, involuntarily, in response to a sudden sound it may be possible, by ignoring most of what has happened, and lopping and trimming the rest to give some sort of semblance to the theory as an explanation of my movement. But suppose I turn my head to look at the time, what corresponds to the receptor side of the voluntary act ? In actual fact nobody has ever succeeded in applying the reflex theory to cortical activity ; and the absurdities of the attempts to do so will be evident in the next chapter.

It was almost exactly a century ago that the idea of reflex action was clarified and the term ' reflex ' introduced by Dr Marshall Hall to describe actions which were limited to the spinal cord and medulla. (16) His conclusions were based on the results of experiments on decapitated snakes, turtles and frogs ; and he was most careful to point out the differences between reflex and other neural functions. Some of the facts concerning reflex activity were already known, but it was not distinguished from other physiological functions. It is the great merit of Marshall Hall that he analysed out this activity from all others. He was careful to exclude from its ambit all voluntary movements, instincts, sensation and rhythmic action ; and to restrict it to such movements as involve only the cord and medulla oblongata. If his successors had been as careful as he, and had shewn his insight into neural action, the science of psychology would have made more rapid strides. The importance of his work justifies a long quotation.

" This property is characterized by being *excited* in its action, and reflex in its course : in every instance in which it is exerted, an impression made upon the extremities of certain nerves is conveyed to the medulla oblongata or the medulla spinalis, and is reflected along other nerves to parts adjacent to, or remote from, that which has received the impression.

" It is by this reflex character that the function to which I have alluded is to be distinguished from every other. There are, in the animal economy, four modes of muscular action. The first is that designated *voluntary* : volition originating in the cerebrum, and spontaneous in its acts, extends its influence along the spinal marrow and the motor nerves, in a *direct line*, to the voluntary muscles. The second is that of *respiration* : like volition, the motive influence in respiration passes in a direct line from one point of the nervous system to certain muscles ; . . . like the voluntary motions, the motions of respiration are spontaneous. The third kind of muscular action in the animal economy is that termed *involuntary* : it depends on the principle of irritability, and requires the *immediate* application of a stimulus to the nervo-muscular fibre itself. . . . There is a fourth which subsists, in part, after the voluntary and respiratory motions have ceased, by the removal of the cerebrum and medulla oblongata, and which is attached to the medulla spinalis, ceasing itself when this is removed, and leaving the irritability undiminished. In this kind of muscular motion, the motive influence does not originate in any central part of the nervous system, but at a distance from that centre : it is neither spontaneous in its action, nor direct in its course ; it is, on the contrary, *excited* by the application of appropriate stimuli, which are not, however, applied immediately to the muscular or nervo-muscular fibre, but to certain membranous parts, whence the impression is carried to the medulla, *reflected*, and reconducted to the part impressed, or conducted to a part remote from it, in which muscular contraction is effected."

Here we have the sphere of reflex action carefully delimited, the term introduced, and its distinction from other nervous acts pointed out. Marshall Hall was also aware that reflex actions are integrated (17) or, as he said, " concatenated as nearly to resemble acts of volition ", by means of which " each and every part of the spinal system is bound in a bond of action with each and every other part of that system." The purposiveness of reflex activity also struck him and he observed that " if the sphincter ani of the frog be irritated, a movement of the posterior extremities, *apparently* designed to remove that irritation, occurs " (his italics). If an object be placed in the hand of a sleeping child it is grasped firmly by means of reflex action. Such phenomena raise the interesting question of the relation of reflex to voluntary action ; and he very acutely pointed out that the former co-operate with the latter. For, if it were otherwise, volition might be opposed or obstructed by reflex activity. In other words reflexes are the servants of volition. We may say that a man makes use of his reflexes, not that they make use of him. The distinction between reflex activity and other action is also shewn by cases of hemiplegia. For, as Hall was aware, and as is now a matter of common knowledge an emotional state can bring an organ into activity when the reflexes are abolished. Of the power of voluntary action in this connection we have previously had examples and more will be found in the next chapter. Again, though it may not be possible to exert any influence voluntarily on the sphincter ani muscles a powerful emotion, such as fear, may cause them to relax.

A curious fate overtook the concept of reflex activity so carefully marked out as we have seen above. The terminology caught on immediately and reflex action finally swallowed up, in its devouring maw, every other sort of nervous functioning. Owing to hasty and unwarranted generalization the very things that Hall was careful to exclude on good and sufficient grounds were all included in the reflex concept.

The wide sweep which has been given to the term is pure dogma, and is simply an attempt to explain living activity on mechanical principles ; since it is assumed that reflex action is easily reducible to mechanics. The complexity of the cortex and the activities which are involved in its working are supposed to be removed if we have simple reflex units to work with. This is done by simply ignoring all action which is not of the reflex pattern. For instance, the secretion of glands may be brought about reflexly, but it can also be brought about by stimulating the gland directly. Again, the distinctive features of spinal reflexes are their invariability and their inevitability. But neither of these characters is found in action dependent on the cortex, for, as we shall see, the results of stimulating cortical points are very variable and by no means inevitable. Moreover, there are certain rhythmic activities such as breathing or heart action which are centrally initiated and not due to distant stimuli.

Thus, on purely physiological grounds, there is no reason for extending the concept of reflex action to all biological activity and the onus of proving that they are reflex rests on those who call them reflex. In fact it would not be going too far to assert that there is no reason for calling cortical activity reflex except that physiologists and psychologists want simple units to work with. Conditioned reflexes have some of the characters of reflex action but differ fundamentally in the fact that they depend on training, and therefore the extension of the term to them is not strictly justified. Moreover, we have shewn that this mode of action is dependent throughout on psychological concepts and is therefore removed from the sphere of reflex action. On all these grounds it is high time that the notion of reflex action is restricted to the sphere to which it rightly belongs and excluded from all others. More especially, in dealing with voluntary action, we must not try to square our explanations of the causal factor in such activity with the dogma that since true reflex action always requires a nervous stimulus, therefore voluntary action must be subject to the same limitation.

Some recent experimental work by K. S. Lashley and Miss J. Ball (18) has thrown doubt on the reflex theory even as an explanation of learning at the perceptual level. The current view of habit-formation is that it consists in forming a series of movements in which the final stages of one movement act as the stimulus to the next ; that in fact a habit is a chain reflex in which each link is the stimulus to the neighbouring one. By this theory it is hoped to get a mechanical view of the nature of habit ; an automatic chain which is self-regulating. Now in the experiments, to which we have referred, all the anatomical tracts in the spinal cord of some rats were severed. The surprising result was obtained that the capacity of the animals to orient themselves and to retain a maze habit was not destroyed. This was the case although the so-called motor-tracts were completely severed ; and the sensory tracts also destroyed. Hence it follows that the explanation of a habit as a series of reflexes each arousing the next is unfounded. If then, even habit-formation does not depend on fixed reflexes it seems preposterous to explain higher activities in terms of the reflex theory. Lashley, whose brilliant work has served to upset all mechanical explanations, still hankers, strangely enough, after a neural basis for habit-formation and would place it tentatively in " some central organization." But it seems much more in consonance with the facts to throw overboard all explanations in terms of physiology and to substitute causal psychological concepts in their place. Such psychological forces can, as we have abundantly shewn, make use of any mechanism which happens to have survived experimental destruction.

CHAPTER IV

PHYSIOLOGICAL PSYCHOLOGY—HUMAN

Now that we have dealt with the results of cerebral injury in the lower animals we may turn to the effects of such injuries in man. However instructive observations on animals may be, it is only when we deal with cerebral lesions in human beings that we can hope to get direct light on the mind-body problem ; for only man is capable of introspection. The study of aphasia provides the most immediate data for this topic, and the history of the development of the concept of aphasia furnishes the most illuminating commentary on the problem. We can trace exactly how the assumptions considered in the first chapter have helped to distort the facts, owing to the attempt to make the facts fit the preconceived ideas. The history of the doctrine of aphasia shews how speculative physiology has served all along to mislead observation and to darken counsel. What happened was this. The majority of psychologists of the nineteenth century believed in an atomic psychology according to which all mental life was built up on the basis of discrete units of sensations, images, ideas, etc. Complex mental states were simply aggregates of these simpler states ; or sometimes the mental atoms were conceived as forming compounds after the analogy of chemical reactions. Physiologists accepted this psychology blindly, and attempted to find evidence for it in the brain. Now the brain consists of cells and fibres, so that it was not difficult to find a ready formed basis for the supposed mental units of sensation, movement, and association. The psychologists having misled the physiologists, were in turn misled by them, and were given distorted clinical observations in support of their erroneous theories. In considering the topic of aphasia we are helped by the masterly study of Dr Henry Head and the account here given is largely indebted to his treatise. (1)

Until the end of the eighteenth century the brain was regarded as a single organ from which animal spirits according to Descartes, or vibrations according to Hartley, passed down to the nerves and controlled bodily actions. At the beginning of the nineteenth century Gall first suggested the idea that the brain consisted of a number of distinct organs subserving different faculties, a view which rapidly led to the absurdities of phrenology. As a result of Gall's work the question of cerebral localization of functions came to the fore, and by the middle of the century the air was full of discussions on this topic. In 1861 Broca, a distinguished anatomist, gave an account of an aphasic patient, *i.e.* of a man who had lost the power of speech but who had retained the general faculty of language. He could hear, understand, and make significant gestures but could not articulate. Subsequent autopsy of this, and of other similar cases, revealed destruction of the inferior frontal convolution of the left side of the brain, since known as Broca's convolution. This discovery opened the flood-gate of nervous ' centres '. There were soon centres for speech, writing, reading and so forth, and destruction of these centres produced aphasia, agraphia, alexia and so on. The idea was that each centre was formed of a group of cells which constituted a specific organ for the corresponding faculty. Centres multiplied rapidly, for speech can be originated both by auditory and visual impressions, so there had to be centres for visual speech, for auditory speech and so on.

It was in vain to try and stem the tide of centres as Hughlings-Jackson, a London physician, attempted to do. Since persons could read and write, and since the brain was the organ of the mind, it was perfectly obvious to all the doctors and psychologists of the period that there must be appropriate centres for these activities in the brain. The sole problem was to locate them in the various convolutions. To Hughlings-Jackson belongs the great merit of realizing that the problem of aphasia and kindred disorders was a psychological one, and that the physiology and anatomy were secondary considerations. The blunder made in attempting to localize language or any other function in certain con volutions was due to the fallacy of over-simplification. Language was regarded as a simple entity, like the movement of a finger. But language is no such simple process. On the contrary it is so extremely complicated that no universally recognized analysis of its structure has yet been made.

Before such an analysis could be attempted it would be necessary to unravel the tangled threads of intellectual and emotional factors which the use of language involves. If we omit to do this, and consider language as a single function, we shall be completely nonplussed when we learn from physicians that ' speechless ' patients can sometimes swear. As swearing is an emotional response it is obvious that some words can be used in one psychological atmosphere but not in another. We can easily realize the mental significance of this observation when we remember that most people would find it difficult, if not impossible, to utter a flippant remark during a religious service. Closely connected with this is the often repeated observation that aphasics are sometimes unable to utter words in one context, or at one time, which they can pronounce in another context or at another time. Thus, one of Dr Head's patients was almost completely speechless, but could reply correctly to questions by saying ' yes ' or ' no '. When asked, however, to utter the word ' yes ' he replied ' No, I can't ' ; and told to repeat the word ' no ' he usually shook his head, but on one occasion he said, ' No, I don't know how to do it '. Anybody who thinks that language can be interpreted in terms of brain processes will have to invent a peculiar kind of neurology to explain this and similar well-attested observations.

Again, language does not consist primarily of words, but of relations expressed between them, that is of propositions. It has become a commonplace to say that, in so far as thought involves language, the proposition is the unit of thinking. This implies that the various words which compose the proposition have their significance entirely determined by the manner in which they are related to each other. If a person were devoid of the language faculty he would be unable to understand a proposition ; yet many ' speechless ' patients understand perfectly well what is said to them, and can communicate their thoughts by pantomime or other methods, without having the ability to utter them. Accordingly, Hughlings-Jackson asserted that the disability known as aphasia, brought on by a brain lesion, was a lack of the power to formulate propositions, a purely psychological incapacity. We may go further than he did and emphasize the fact that the essential factor in language is word-value and that the aphasic's disabilities are largely due to a loss of the appreciation of such values. If I contemplate a picture or listen to a symphony it is simple matter to state where the picture is situated, or the place where the orchestra is playing, but it would be perfectly meaningless to enquire as to the locus of their æsthetic value. This seems to me analogous to the query with regard to the localization of the function of language. Much of the theory of cerebral localization is due to the misleading implications of terminology. A name is given to some particular function, such as language, and the simplicity and unity of the name is held to imply a corresponding unity and simplicity of function.

The history of science is full of cases in which observed facts are unconsciously twisted and distorted by experts to make them fit into preconceived theories. Thus it came about that the prevailing psychological atmosphere caused Hughlings-Jackson's work to be neglected until Head resuscitated it, and the searchers after brain ' centres ' had it all their own way. The belief that all the operations of the intellect could only be understood in terms of nerve cells and fibres held the field. Now, words can be both read and heard, and consequently disorders of speech must be due to destruction of visual and auditory centres, or to the obstruction of the paths between such centres, or from them to the organs of speech. Hence arose a school of diagram-makers who shewed exactly what happened in the brain by geometrical drawings. Such pictures became the standards by which cases of aphasia or kindred diseases were investigated ; and the clinical forms of disordered function were deduced as rigorously from them as from a geometrical proposition. If an unfortunate patient exhibited symptoms which could not be interpreted by the diagrams, the former were ignored or twisted about, so as to make the case correspond with a lesion of some cortical centre or hypothetical pathway. The autopsies did not reveal the suspected lesions, but so much the worse for the autopsies, for the diagrams could not err. Psychologists had an easy time, for acting on the assumption that all mental phenomena consist solely of sensory and motor processes combined by the law of association, it was perfectly simple to explain memory by a diagram. Each fact remembered was indicated by a circle which represented a brain centre, and its association with other facts by straight lines between them which represented association fibres. The psychology of reasoning was dealt with in the same fashion. In order to reason we must, of course, have data, which must be connected in some way. What is easier than to represent the former by circles and the connections by straight lines. As no man was killed immediately after he remembered something or had performed a process of reasoning, there was no direct means of confirming or refuting the theory by a post-mortem examination. The diagrams, therefore, settled the matter ; they were drawn and the facts must somehow or other fit into the scheme.

After Broca's discovery the next important step in cerebral localization was taken by Fritsch and Hitzig, who in the year 1870 discovered the ' motor area '. By stimulating certain points in the cortex they were able to produce isolated movements of certain muscles. Thenceforward, by an astonishing flight of logic, the motor area was regarded as the seat of the function of separate voluntary movements and of volition in general. Shortly afterwards H. Munk determined the position of the visual areas in the occipital lobes, as injury to these was thought to lead to permanent blindness. Subsequently an auditory area was mapped out in the temporal lobe, and it was considered that the functions of these various areas were sharply delimited. These discoveries, combined with the dogma of a point-to-point correspondence between mental

F

events and neural processes, were held to demand a rigid localization of function in the brain.

Now this view is startling even on purely anatomical considerations, and shews how a firmly held theory may blind us to the most obvious facts. For, as we saw previously, the so-called association fibre system places all parts of the cortex in intimate physiological connection. An isolated cortical centre is, therefore, a monstrosity. Owing to its structure, the essential feature of cortical activity is the correlation and integration of nervous impulses. The disturbance of the state of physiological equilibrium of the cortex by an incoming set of impulses may reverberate to the extreme limits, if the chronaxies are suitably adjusted ; and it is a mere abstraction to consider the parts of the brain in isolation from each other.

At the beginning of this century P. Marie attacked the whole received doctrine of cerebral localization in aphasia, on psychological grounds, insisting that aphasics suffered primarily from defects of the intellectual operations associated with the use of language. When the intelligence is intact, inability to talk (anarthria) may exist without much interference with the other uses of language, such as comprehension of speech, reading silently and writing. Clinical observations are not conclusive ; since what a patient is suffering from seems to depend to a considerable extent on who is examining him, and the general emotional atmosphere surrounding him. Thus as Dr Head states " familiar surroundings, friendly people, sympathetic handling and the mode of examination have a profound effect on the results obtained." And all these are psychological considerations which have nothing to do with brain lesions. Similarly, when a counsel browbeats a witness he may cause him to forget or distort certain facts, without in any way interfering with his brain mechanisms.

The distinction between the psychological point of view and the physiological is well brought out by the consideration of certain other disorders of function which are closely akin to aphasia. There is a condition known as *apraxia*, in which a person is unable to move various parts of the body such as an arm or leg, although there is no motor paralysis, or sensory disability. The man has an intact sensori-motor apparatus, but cannot employ it to carry out what he wants to do ; more especially is he disabled from those habitual activities acquired by experience. The anatomical organs are sound, but the psychological processes cannot make use of them. Thus an apraxic patient might be able to walk when he is paying no particular attention to the process, but quite incapable of obeying an order to walk across the room. It has been suggested that motor aphasia is but an instance of apraxia affecting the speech organs. But we cannot express a high grade activity, such as the use of language, in terms of units of muscular movement. An activity, such as speech, is no more made up of atomic units of muscular movement than a complex mental activity is composed of mental units. Speech is a unitary whole and to attempt to analyse it into its component movements is about as sensible as the attempt to describe a picture as consisting of so many separate square inches of different coloured paint.

Corresponding to apraxia on the practical side of mental life, there is a disorder brought about by gross brain lesions called *agnosia*, which is a defect of the receptive side of consciousness. Agnosia may take a variety of forms, visual, auditory or tactile. In all these cases sensory impressions cannot be properly interpreted. A patient suffering from visual agnosia, for example, may be able to see such an object as a chair and avoid it when walking, but he may not be able to recognize its legs or say what is their use. But, though he may not be able to recognize an object when presented to his vision, he may find no difficulty in recognition if he is allowed to handle it. He may be able to see a printed page, but find it utterly impossible to interpret the symbols, and consequently to read. Nevertheless his power of writing the same words may not be affected. A man suffering from auditory agnosia will be similarly afflicted with regard to his hearing. Here again the disorder, though due to a lesion, is primarily psychical and cannot even be described in sensory terms, but only in terms of functional psychology.

The attempt has frequently been made to describe all the

above varieties of imperception as being due to the loss of images, owing to the destruction of cerebral tissue in which they are located. It has been said that the reason the patient cannot recognize the chair is because he has lost the visual images which he has stored up ; and these are necessary to give meaning to the sensory impression. But, where introspection is possible, it can be shewn that the man has not lost his images and he may be quite well able to imagine a chair. What he has lost is a certain mental capacity to read meaning into his images and impressions. It must always be borne in mind that a mental image, like a sensation, is an abstraction and only exists as part of a complete psychical act and never in isolation. Consciousness has happily been compared by William James to a stream. " The traditional psychology talks like one who should say a river consists of nothing but pailsful, spoonsful, quartpotsful, barrelsful, and other moulded forms of water. Even were the pails and the pots all actually standing in the stream, still between them the free water would continue to flow. Every definite image in the mind is steeped and dyed in the free water that flows round it. With it goes the sense of its relations, near and remote, the dying echo of whence it came to us, the dawning sense of whither it is to lead. The significance, the value, of the image is all in this halo or penumbra that surrounds and escorts it . . . or rather that is fused into one with it and has become bone of its bone and flesh of its flesh." If this is sound psychology, as it undoubtedly is, it is futile to attempt to find a locality for images in some specific region of the cortex, or to consider them as stored up, like so many photographic negatives, in particular brain centres. Rather we may say, that in so far as the brain is involved in conscious processes, every particular act of thought calls into play the whole cerebral mechanism. Moreover, as we have already suggested and shall see in detail in a later chapter, the whole idea of mental images being stored up in the brain, or dependent on nervous functioning is a myth.

It should be obvious, now, that the attempt to localize any vital process in a centre is due to a variety of causes.

First there is the assumption that mental events can only be understood as the reflections of brain events. Then there is the notion of a point-to-point correspondence between the two series of events ; and, since the brain can be divided up into a congeries of different areas, it is assumed that the mental events are capable of a similar analysis. Connected with this was the widespread belief in atomic mental events, which we have just seen to be devoid of any foundation. Finally there is the influence of terminology leading to inadequate clinical diagnosis. Thus, if we define aphasia as loss of speech, it is fatally easy to consider it as a single thing and to adjust our observations accordingly. But loss of speech may take a variety of forms, and no two cases of aphasia are alike. Two patients, for example, may be unable to give names to everyday objects, yet one of them may be able to pick out the appropriate names from printed slips whilst the other is unable to do this. Another, whilst incapable of naming objects, such as colours, may be able to describe them, referring to black, for instance, as ' what you wear for the dead '.

Sometimes, as the result of cerebral injury, a man loses the ability to write, described clinically as *agraphia*. Now, the mere giving of a name to this disturbance of function is apt to be very misleading. Agraphia and similar terms are far too abstract, and when applied to concrete cases are most inadequate. A man suffering from ' agraphia ' can sometimes write his name when combined with his address, but not in isolation. To understand this it is essential to pay attention to the psychological situation as a whole, that is to the configuration with which the man is confronted, and not merely to the elements into which the situation may be analysed by an observer. The inability to separate out one item of a complete configuration may be combined with the power to reproduce the situation as a whole. We have here an example of the error referred to in an earlier chapter, namely the carrying over into psychology of terminology borrowed from physiology. An electrical stimulus may produce an isolated movement in an excised muscle, but there is nothing in human behaviour corresponding to an isolated stimulus determining conduct. The pattern of behaviour does not correspond to the pattern of stimuli in a presented situation. What a person reacts to is the total meaning of a situation, and not to the abstract elements into which a psychologist can analyse the configuration. The interpretation and analysis of psychological processes from the physiological standpoint merely leads to confusion. A reflex act, for example, can readily be analysed into two main portions, a receptive phase or the so-called sensory side, and a reactive phase, the motor aspect. When this analysis is combined with the assumption that all neural activity, including that of the brain, is of the reflex type, it is a short step to the belief that mental process can be analysed into sensations and movements.

But such a function as that of speech cannot be understood in sensory and motor terms. For, as Head has rightly pointed out, language is based on complex integrated functions " standing higher in the neural hierarchy than motion or sensation, and when it is disturbed, the clinical manifestations appear in terms of these complex *psychical* processes ; they cannot be classed under *physiological* categories, motor or sensory, nor even under such headings as visual and auditory " (italics mine). No analysis of speech in terms of simple physiological processes can explain why an aphasic, as frequently happens, succeeds in speaking under certain conditions but fails altogether under a different set of circumstances. Nevertheless, Dr S. A. Kinnier Wilson (2) who is well aware of the psychological nature of speech, cannot rid himself of the belief that words are sensory and motor units whose images or engrams are in some mysterious fashion ' stored ' in the brain. This leads him to invent all sorts of centres, located where they ought to be from the clinical standpoint. He does admit, however, that " some day, perhaps, knowledge of clinico-anatomical cerebral localization will be sufficiently advanced to justify its use as a basis for aphasic classification, but at present the data are still incomplete ". If, however, the clinician is searching for data to account for the atomic constituents of consciousness, namely isolated words or images, we can safely say that he will never find them, since he is looking for the physiological substratum of the non-existent. A pianist cannot play properly if some of the strings of the piano are broken, but it would be absurd to try to discover the cause of correct playing by examining the mechanism of the piano.

It must be evident from the facts we have adduced that aphasia and kindred disorders of speech cannot be explained, or even described, in neurological terms. In order to interpret such disorders we must make use of psychological concepts ; and this is the view that Dr Head and others have taken as the result of the examination of a large number of cases of aphasia due to unilateral injuries of the brain sustained in the war. His diagnoses were based on a number of carefully graded tests ; for it is only by graduation that an analysis of the defect is possible. His conclusion is that such disorders are due to an inability to employ or interpret symbols correctly. Between the initiation of an act and its execution there usually intervenes some sort of symbol, verbal or otherwise. Thus, if I have an appointment I look at my watch, the face of which is a symbolic representation of the passage of time ; or I may consult my diary, in which case verbal symbols are interposed. The power to interpret or employ symbolism is entirely a psychical process. It consists in the ability to disregard the sense-elements in an experience, and to pay attention solely to the implied meanings. Regarded from this standpoint the paradoxical difficulties to which we previously alluded, where words and expressions may be used in one context but not in another, need no longer perplex us. For the meaning of exactly the same symbol may be totally changed when the context is changed.

Looked at from the point of view of symbolic thinking and expression, disturbances of language, due to an unilateral lesion of the cortex, may assume a variety of forms, and are classified by Dr Head under four categories. It must be borne in mind that it is not speech alone but that writing and other symbolic modes of expression may be affected by brain lesions. There are first of all *verbal* defects, in which the patient cannot find the word he requires, either for utterance or for silent thinking. It is the actual structural formulation of the word which is missing, not the comprehension of its meaning; since the sufferer can sometimes select the word from a series of printed cards, though he cannot form it for himself. The second category of defects comprises what are known as *nominal* defects, since the deficiency consists in a want of comprehension of the nominal value of words or other symbols. There may be no difficulty in articulating words or phrases, but the words do not fit the objects to which the man wishes to refer. In a Montessori school one of the exercises a child has to perform is to fit various geometrical forms into their appropriate insets in a board. Persons suffering from nominal defects cannot, as it were, choose the correct verbal forms to fit into the meaning they intend. Sometimes they can indicate what they mean by making use of a descriptive phrase instead of the word. Thus one patient who could not name the time of day referred to a particular hour, correctly, as " the time when you eat ". In the third form of defect, called *syntactical*, the man is able to form words but he mixes them all up, and consequently talks jargon. He can understand the meaning of what he reads, but cannot read it intelligibly to others. Finally there are *semantic* defects. Just as a child below the age of six cannot describe a picture but merely enumerates the items it contains, so those who suffer from semantic defects are unable to combine into a single whole a series of relevant details. They have no difficulty in naming objects, or uttering words, nor is their syntax thrown out of gear ; but they have lost the power to combine details into a coherent scheme. When they read a story, for example, they may take in all the points but miss the point.

The existence of these varieties of disorders of speech shews how misleading it is to describe aphasia as a loss of the function of speech : and to localize the function in a restricted region of the brain is to over-simplify a complex process by subsuming totally different phenomena under a single name. Again, the physiological standpoint is quite inappropriate, even for descriptive purposes. Verbal aphasia, for example, may exist without any paralysis of the lips and tongue, and nominal aphasia without any interference with vision. That is to say, the physiological mechanism may be quite adequate for some particular purpose but cannot be used for some other purpose. If we may make use of a loose analogy, it is as though a typewriter invariably produced English sentences but never French. In that case it would be futile to say that the machine could not type French. The lack of function would naturally be sought in the ignorance of the typist of the French language. Similarly, in aphasia, the inability to exercise some function does not reside in the mechanism, but in some mental incapacity which must be investigated by psychological methods. And we must never forget, in this connection, that the loss of function in aphasia is not absolute but relative ; for a patient who cannot speak or read under certain conditions, may be able to do so if the task is presented to him in some other way.

It should be evident from what has been said that aphasia is not a single functional defect which can be assumed to have its seat in a definite brain centre or centres. The term is a shorthand description for a variety of abnormal modes of behaviour comprising phenomena of very various origin. Speech is the response to certain situations, and use is made of mechanisms which are under the control of the person as the result of prolonged experience. Aphasia shews the attempt of a person to meet certain situations with physiological or psychological mechanisms which are defective in some way ; and its varieties shew the manner in which these defects are met. If it were simply a question of a function located in a centre or centres those cases, to which we have referred, in which a patient can overcome his disability, in a more or less ingenious indirect way, would be quite unintelligible ; for the destruction of the centre ought to destroy the function. Again, as has been previously mentioned, an aphasic patient who is described as speechless may, under the stress of emotion, give vent to his feelings by swearing. Thus he is not essentially wordless, but what he lacks is the voluntary control over words. In proportion as a task demands a high degree of symbolic formulation and expression, in that proportion is the task difficult for an aphasic. For instance, he may not be able to read the time from a clock but he may be able to reproduce the time on another clock face, for this latter task is mere copying, and the symbolic part of the process is reduced to a minimum. Finally, it must be remembered that anxiety or worry may profoundly affect the ability of an aphasic to cope with verbal expressions. As these emotional states affect normal people in the same way, so that when a man is greatly distressed he makes many verbal blunders, it will be easily understood that the processes concerned in the function of language are mainly psychical and not physiological. The same is true of other functions usually considered as dependent on the body, namely habit, memory, instinct, etc. These, likewise, are thrown out of gear when a man is for any reason mentally distracted. Even the most expert player plays games badly when in a state of anxiety.

We may now attempt to unravel the tangled web of facts so far considered in order to smooth out the mind-body problem. Two clues are immediately suggested as starting points, namely the doctrine of ' centres ' and the associated theory of the ' localization of function ' in the brain. Centres are supposed to be specially restricted groups of cells initiating and carrying out some specific function, which is consequently assumed to be localized in that region. The existence of such centres is supposed to be established, as we have indicated, by two sets of observations ; first the results obtained by electrically stimulating different parts of the ' motor area ', and secondly the clinical observations that differently localized brain lesions produce different disturbances of function.

Now, more exact experiment has shewn that the response obtained from stimulating the same point in the motor cortex is by no means constant, but varies, both as regards the kind of movement and the organ moved. Two successive stimulations of the same point in the cortex may produce first extension and then flexion of the same finger joints. Again, the movement produced by stimulating any point depends on the preceding events in the brain. Thus when the successive points of the motor area were stimulated, from above downwards, until the region was reached where the response was a flexion of the elbow, it was found that by reversing the process, and proceeding from below upwards, that stimulating the same region produced movements of the thumb and index finger. It has even been found that stimulation of the elbow region may, at another time, produce facial movements. It is evident that the motor cortex is a very labile region and it is consequently incorrect to regard it as the seat of strictly limited centres of pre-ordained functions. The response from any particular area depends on what has previously happened, and, in turn, determines what will happen in the future. This makes it misleading to speak of 'centres' for definite movements, and, more particularly, to think of speech movements as 'localized' in a definite region. And the facts considered in the last chapter amply confirm this view.

If we leave aside for a moment the fact that language is primarily a psychical function, and concentrate our attention solely on the speech movements, it would be a blunder to regard these as composed of a series of isolated acts. For speech, like every other function consists of an orderly, co-ordinated, and highly integrated march of events. As all parts of the brain are interconnected, the impulses producing the co-ordinated speech movements must run through the nervous system like water through a complicated system of pipes. A break in the system produces a functional disorder, as the impulses are temporarily blocked ; but some other part of the brain will, sooner or later, be found, which renders the function possible in a modified form, as the observations of the last chapter have so conclusively demonstrated.

Like every other frequently repeated function, spoken language tends to become more and more automatic. The automatism depends in an increasing degree on the co-ordinated sequence of a series of predetermined reactions. A brain lesion disturbs this orderly sequence, but even if the whole 'centre' is destroyed the process can be relearnt. We may, therefore, think of a centre as a region where the progress of some co-ordinated activity can be inhibited, deviated or reinforced. The cortex may be regarded as an organ whereby our automatic activities can be modified at will, but in no sense an organ where they are independently initiated. A functional activity, such as language, cannot be destroyed by brain injury, since the function is mental. The loss supervening on brain injuries is only a deviation of function, for as we have said, a man who cannot read or write owing to a lesion on the left side of the brain, can sometimes do so if the task is presented to him in a new way. And, as we have shewn before and shall see more fully later, he may be able under suitable conditions completely to recover his lost ability.

If the brain only has the function we have assigned to it, the question may be raised as to why a lesion may produce such profound effects, even if these are only temporary. The answer is to be sought in the lowered state of vitality of the organism as a whole as the result of any injury. When the spinal cord of a man is seriously injured, for instance, the lower limbs become flaccid and all deep reflexes are abolished. But as the shock passes away, especially in a healthy man, the reflexes appear once more and, in fact, are more easily excitable. In a similar fashion our acquired automatic acts are interfered with by anything which diminishes our general well being. When we are feeling ' out of sorts ' our movements become listless, our walk loses its spring, we play games badly, and even our speech may shew signs of disturbance. It must also be remembered that the nature of the loss of function brought about by a brain injury is largely determined by the severity and acuteness of the lesion rather than by its *locus*. The general lowered vitality is, therefore, adequate to explain loss of function, without any need to suppose that functions are, strictly speaking, localized in any part of the cortex.

Enough has been said to shew that the mind-body problem is distorted if we approach it from the physiological side. The necessity for the psychological approach is well brought out by a consideration of those disorders of speech in which certain phrases are retained when they no longer have any significance for thought. There are certain linguistic expressions which have become as automatic as the process of walking ; such every-day phrases or locutions as ' listen to me ', ' I tell you that ', ' what I mean is ', etc., etc. Closely allied to these are interjections, swear words, and other words expressive of emotion. In cases of aphasia these automatic locutions may be retained whilst the patient loses the power of significant speech, *i.e.* the power of employing symbols to express ideas. What is lost is a psychical activity, whilst what remains, though it has the outward form of language, is as little mental as the act of tying one's shoes. This is the psychological explanation of the curious fact, previously mentioned, and totally inexplicable in physiological terms, that an aphasic person may be quite unable to employ a particular word in a significant phrase though he has still the power to utter that word. An instructive example is given by Dr S. A. Kinnier Wilson (2) of one of his patients " who suffered from motor aphasia in the ordinary sense and saw a Zeppelin descend in flames one night on the outskirts of London and ejaculated ' Hallelujah ! ' under the stress of his emotion, which word he has never since been able to repeat ' propositionally '." In so far as the word is a significant symbol the man's power to use it is lost, but inasmuch as it is a mere emotional expression he may be able to say it. A similar conclusion is indicated by the relation of feeling to language capacity. It is a matter of common observation that strong emotion sometimes interferes with the free use of language, and some emotions aid it. The great majority of people are unable to express themselves in the face of an audience. In other words, an emotion can temporarily produce the same effects as a brain lesion. And Dr Head's clinical observations led him to the conclusion that " Both the power and mode of expression are profoundly affected by the relation of the patient to his auditor. One person can help an aphasic, whilst another produces an inhibitory effect, even on his capacity to think." Everybody can confirm these observations from his own daily experience of normal people. In brief, what an aphasic suffers from depends very largely on who it is that examines him ; and the conclusion strongly suggested is that the disability is primarily a mental one.

If we take a wide survey of the part played by language in the process of thinking, we soon realize that its main purpose is to release us from the bonds of sense perception. For language enables us to manipulate relations of every kind, spatial, temporal, logical, etc., independently of the terms so related. Again the use of language eliminates the cruder form of trial and error. Thus, if I have to fit together the pieces of a jig-saw puzzle I am guided entirely by perception, and make use of trial and error ; whereas if I deal with geometrical insets I can at once pick out the triangular, the circular or other pieces from a large number of shapes and fit them into appropriate places by the help of the correct nomenclature. Moreover, the systematic analysis of the properties of any object depends entirely on the use of words, which make possible the selection of certain aspects or relationships, and the ignoring of others. It would hardly be feasible, for example, to distinguish the various aspects of a colour, such as tone, saturation, purity, etc., unless symbols had been invented for the purpose. Where words are lacking, as in the case of taste or smell, the corresponding sensations cannot be fully analysed. Finally, it is not possible to see how any form of generalization could be achieved without the use of abstract terms and symbols. Certainly mathematics would not be possible without them. Now all the above-named processes are more or less disturbed in the different varieties of aphasia ; all of them depend on the correct use of symbolism ; and all are mental.

With the facts now at our disposal we may now consider what peculiar part, if any, the cerebral cortex plays in mental life. It is the most fundamental postulate of physiological psychology that the essential immediate condition of all consciousness is the activity of the cortex. In the light of what we have already learnt we must interpret this postulate in a very vague way. For, as we have discarded the theory of fixed ' centres ', there can be no point-to-point correspondence between any mental function, such as language, and the activity of some definite group of nerve cells. Now, when a cortical lesion disturbs some particular function it often happens that the man reverts to some more primitive mode of accomplishing the same end. In the variety of aphasia, previously called ' nominal ', there is an inability to comprehend the nominal value of words or other symbols. For instance, if a number is uttered to the patient he fails to recognize its significance ; or the name of a day of the week may convey no meaning to him. If, however, he is allowed to count on his fingers, or go through the names of the days of the week in a serial order, he slowly realizes the meanings of these words. The patient proceeds exactly as a young child does. What he suffers from is not the loss of the psychical function, but inability to react on a certain level. The level of the function is depressed, as it were, to a more primitive height ; just as a child cannot be said to have no power of reasoning, but simply reasons at a lower level. The power of reasoning does not arise at a definite point of time, but rather becomes more and more perfect with the lapse of time. A cortical injury, therefore, does not abolish a function, but forces the person to carry out the activity in some other, and usually, more primitive fashion. High grade functioning at the human level is a process of slow growth. It is not surprising, then, to find cases of human injury to the cortex in which, unlike the lower animals, the function appears to be completely lost ; since the time for restitution may be insufficient to regain the human level, or the will to recover may be lacking.

When, however, the will to recover is sufficiently strong, a function may be resumed which has apparently been completely lost as the result of a cerebral lesion. An instructive instance of such restitution of function is furnished by the case of a medical man, Dr Saloz (3) who was suddenly attacked with aphasia at the age of sixty years, and subsequently wrote an account of his own case. The autopsy shewed a considerable atrophy of the left hemisphere especially in the ' speech area ' (Broca's convolution) both in the cortical and sub-cortical regions ; the latter being soft and almost diffluent. At the outset of the attack he had complete verbal aphasia except for a few expressions of an automatic kind, such as ' no ', ' yes ', ' thanks '. He could not read the simplest word, or even letters of the alphabet, and had completely lost the power to write. With an ordinary person, at this time of life, there is no doubt that the loss of function would have been permanent, as he would have given up all hope of recovery ; and it would require considerable courage to face the task of learning all over again. For this reason elderly people usually make little progress when attacked by aphasia. But Dr Saloz had an iron will and made up his mind to recover his lost faculties.

He says that he felt at first as one immured in a sepulchre, that he knew what he wished to express, but had lost all the instruments of expression and that symbols conveyed nothing to him. It seemed to him that he had entered another world where his ideas were soft and downy, as in a dream. His thoughts were hazy as though a veil enclosed him. In so far as expression necessitates the use of symbols, he had nothing with which to express himself. He had ideas, thoughts or conceptions, but lacked the symbols of expression. The sense of his thoughts appeared like a far-off echo, which recalled the things, without the intervention of the words. " J'avais donc perdu la mémoire du mot, mais il me restait le souvenir de la place qu'il occupait."

With wonderful determination he set about recovering his lost faculties by a prolonged course of self re-education, to which he devoted all his energies. He proceeded in the manner of a child learning to speak, read and write. Starting with the letters he laboriously worked his way through syllables to words, and at the end of three years of persistent effort had so completely recovered that he was able to write a complete account of his case. His recovery was due, as he himself remarks, to an imperious desire to get back what he had lost, combined with a dogged persistence. Lacking symbols of expression he found it difficult to fix his thoughts. " Quand on m'a dit de prononcer mon nom, je me rapelle très bien que mon nom me disait rien du tout." But by repeated efforts it seemed to come, "comme un echo lointain qui se rapproche de plus en plus, pour aboutir à mon nom effectif, mais qui disparaissait aussitôt comme s'il était voilé tout d'un coup par un espèce de gaze floue."

Cases such as this should make us cautious in accepting evidence about the effects of cerebral injuries. If structure determines function, as most neurologists believe, then the study of the brain should throw some light on mental functioning. But we have seen that this hope had always proved a delusion. Dr Saloz's left hemisphere was extensively atrophied, especially in the ' speech centre ', in the middle of which there was destruction of substance and the sub-cortical parts were almost fluid. There ought, therefore, to have been a permanent loss of the major portion of his ability to use language. If a ' wireless set ' had its valves injured, its wires broken or almost fluid, its connections imperfect, we should not expect it to be efficient in reproducing sounds. Yet, despite the fact that the brain mechanisms never recovered, as was shewn by a subsequent autopsy, Dr Saloz regained his speech and writing so completely that he was able to write his memoirs from which I have quoted, and to study the medical literature of aphasia in order to discuss his own case. Doubtless this was due to the fact that "en tout cas, pour moi, quelque chose emerge des profondeurs de ma pensée, c'est la *volonté* d'aboutir malgré tout ". The only defect that his friend and physician could discover in him, after his recovery, was a certain lack of suppleness, and obstinacy in adhering to his first opinions ! As most of us suffer from these blemishes, most of our lives, there does not seem to have been any permanent loss of function. We may safely conclude that, as far as mind is concerned, its functioning is not, in any intelligible sense, dependent upon brain structure. For when the structure collapses the mind is still able to accomplish its purposes with the wrecked mechanism, provided only that these are sufficiently firmly held. Everything points to some functional organization which can make use of any structure. Lashley gives the following startling example. "In an animal

G

which died during a recent experiment, the entire right hemisphere was found to have been replaced by a purulent cyst, and the left was so softened as to be removed with difficulty from the cranium ; yet on the day of his death this animal made a perfect record in a difficult discrimination test." (4)

The theory of nervous ' centres ' initiating and controlling mental activity must be definitely abandoned. Such centres may subserve a purely physiological function in co-ordinating and integrating nervous impulses, but there is no evidence for the view that centres are fixed or unalterable. Can we, then, in any intelligible sense still continue to speak of the localization of function in the brain ? To answer this question we must consider physiological functioning in general. The separation of the various parts of the body into different organs, with isolated functions, is an artificial abstraction. No organ can be considered in isolation from all the others. Of course we have to study them separately, but this is a methodological device and not an expression of existing facts. Still less can we separate the various portions of the central nervous system. The system is a unity which, at any moment, is in a state of neutral equilibrium. When nervous impulses invade the system the centre of gravity is continually shifting. The amount of shift depends, not only on the incoming impulses but also on the pre-existing state of the rest of the system. (5) To imagine that what is going on in one part could be considered without reference to the concurrent activity of all the others is to ignore the distinguishing feature of brain anatomy, namely the intimate connection brought about by the so-called association fibres. It is quite impossible to suppose that a set of nervous impulses could be restricted to any definitely circumscribed area. Even the chronaxies of the fibres are variable within very wide limits. And, as a matter of direct observation, we know that an injury to any one part of the brain sets up a shock which reverberates to widely spread areas and interferes with all other nervous activity, a phenomenon which has received the name of *diaschisis*.

But we cannot stop at the nervous system. Directly or indirectly all parts of the organism are functionally interwoven. Any activity of one part, in some way or another, must affect the whole of the organism, either through the glands or the common blood supply or through the nervous impulses which all activity sets going. As Dr E. Miller (6), has pithily expressed it : " The study of the nervous system has so far expanded that we know how it influences the very glands themselves, although it never dominates them, the two being always reciprocally related. If these discoveries have torn the nimbus from neurology (the one time government-house of human behaviour), it is not upon the head of endocrinology that the halo has descended. There is no aristocratic organ in the body, the crown is borne by no particular tissue. We have learned to regard the body-mind organization as an organic commonwealth." And moreover, since an organism cannot have any activity apart from its environment, it is a fallacious abstraction to consider it as existing *in vacuo.* Just as we have found it impossible to locate any function in a specific part of the brain, but must consider the nervous system as a whole, and just as we cannot consider the nervous system apart from the rest of the organism, so we now see that we cannot treat the organism apart from its environment. If, then, we are to continue to speak of localization of function, the activity of those parts of the environment which are essential for the activity must also be taken into account ; and all nervous functions are localized both within and without the body. What is not localized in any definite place cannot intelligibly be said to be localized at all.

Professor Haldane (7), who has the great merit of being not only a physiologist but a philosopher, has put this clearly. " When " he says " we examine the physiological activities of the brain we find that it is in constant active connection through afferent nerves with all parts of the body and so with the surrounding environment. A response to an afferent impulse through a sense organ is determined, not merely by the nature and strength of this impulse, but also by the coincident inpouring of impulses from all parts of the body and surrounding environment. . . . A nervous response is also directly dependent on the amount and quality of the blood supply to the nervous system, and thus indirectly on the functional activity of the rest of the organism, and on its relations to the environment through nutrition and respiration. A very slight excess of carbonic acid or deficiency of oxygen has a marked effect on the nervous responses to afferent stimuli ; and immediate loss of consciousness results from great excess or deficiency.

With every advance in physiology the experimental evidence shews more and more clearly that we cannot separate off and specify the occurrences in separate parts of the body, and particularly of the central nervous system, as we can for practical purposes separate off and specify the occurrences in different parts of a machine. In nervous responses, and more particularly in conscious reponses, the whole nervous system, and mediately the whole organism and its environment are involved. The response is a manifestation of the whole life of the organism, and not merely the response of the brain or a definite part of it."

These general considerations receive confirmation from an investigation recently undertaken into the nature of the tests employed to diagnose aphasia. (8) The earlier tests were of the crudest kind being limited to finding out whether a patient could speak, read or write. Dr Head improved the diagnosis by introducing serial tests of a graduated kind. One of these tests consisted in the physician performing certain movements, such as touching his right or left eye or ear with his right or left hand and asking the patient to copy these movements. The test is similar to that of a gymnastic instructor facing a class who have to copy his motions. Of course, the patient has to reverse the seen movements. And it has been maintained that, in order to do this, he must have recourse to internal speech, *i.e.* reproduce mentally in words what the physician is doing. Now the majority of aphasics do this test badly, and in some cases they reverse all the movements, using their right hands instead of their left or vice versa. Such blunders are attributed to a lack of facility in the use of language. But normal people make exactly the same blunders, and it has been proved that mistakes are due to the lack of the power of discriminating and manipulating spatial relations correctly. The ability investigated by such tests is that of spatial orientation ; and other tests of aphasia presuppose the same faculty.

Several aphasics are known to suffer from grave affections of orientation, evidenced by such observations as their inability to find their way about in familiar surroundings or to set out a plan of a familiar room and so on. And it is probable that, if the methods of diagnosis were more detailed, all aphasics would shew similar disorders of spatial perception. Confirmation of this belief has been provided by the work of W. van Woerkom (9) who made a careful study of the restitution of function in one of his aphasic patients. For the first two weeks this man was dumb, but after one month he was able to name objects and thenceforward improved. So complete was his process of re-education that, after six weeks, a superficial observer could have detected nothing abnormal about him except that he expressed himself with difficulty. Nevertheless a careful examination shewed a profound loss of function. He could not place a ruler parallel to another at a short distance, but crossed them fumblingly ; nor could he imitate the directions of a stick moved in the air. With his eyes bandaged he failed to imitate passive movements impressed on his limbs. He could not place an object correctly on one side or another of a stick even if he was shewn what to do. He could point successively to two objects in front of him, but could not indicate their spatial relation either by words or gestures. In fact his geometrical sense was abolished almost completely. He could carry out purely habitual acts, such as lighting a cigar, since these do not involve any idea of the movement to be made, but are secondarily reflex activities. What he lacked was the idea, or representation, of movement.

Now much of our everyday thinking involves the manipulation of spatial ideas which as a result of our education have become unconscious. I agree therefore, with Dr R.

Mourgue (10) that aphasia is but a special case of a more general disturbance of function. This special defect has been long recognized and investigated ; but the more general loss has been overlooked, because not detected clinically. When we come to discuss the psychology of language we shall see that the separation of a language into words is a highly artificial procedure which has only arisen because language was reduced to writing. There is, as we shall see, nothing in spoken speech to correspond to this. In order to reduce the unbroken volume of spoken sound to separate phrases or words a long process of demarcation or differentiation is necessary. Such differentiation or splitting up of a whole into parts lies also at the basis of our spatial discrimination of sensory experiences. So that the elementary psychological processes which underlie spatial perception are also the basis of the analysis of language. Language is disturbed by a cortical lesion for the same reason that spatial orientation is disturbed ; namely that certain elementary psychological processes are rendered more difficult. For exactly the same reason agraphia and other forms of apraxia are also involved. With these considerations in mind it is utterly absurd to suppose that words are in any conceivable sense ' stored up in the brain '. We might as well suppose that space is stored up in the same way, and nobody has ever been foolish enough to suggest this. Before we can accept clinical observations as evidence for the mind-body problem we ought to assure ourselves that clinicians have thoroughly analysed the functions they examine. And we now see that the varieties of aphasia should not be regarded as diseases, but as symptoms of some underlying defects of a psychological nature. Restitution of function, when the injury to the brain is permanent, shews that various parts of the cortex are equipotential in carrying out the psychological function.

We have now completed our survey of the facts of physiology which are supposed to explain mental activity, or, at least, to underlie it. The examination has shewn that, at every single step, there are unfounded assumptions and dogmas. Wherever physiological observations have been brought forward to account for mental states they have proved either erroneous or unnecessary. Mind and body have a unique unity ; a whole which is *sui generis*. We can never hope to get light on the mind-body problem by considering in isolation facts derived from either source. It is in fact impossible to get an answer to the question what is the relation of the mind to the body. For this formulates the question in such a way as to make any answer *ab initio* erroneous. Both the historical answers, namely psycho-physical parallelism and interactionism, presuppose that a separation between mind and body exists in a living organism. But a body animated by a mind is not a corpse animated by a ghost. When the mind leaves the body there has not been anything which can be described as an act of subtraction, but a totally new phenomenon appears. We can as little imagine the resulting corpse acting on a mind, or a mind acting on it, as we can suppose a cunning workman constructing a model of the brain which shall be animated ; though, as we have seen, he could produce a very fair model simulating all the properties of the nervous impulses. The real question is how the unity which we may call the mind-body is related to the person who owns it, and employs it in his dealings with the external world. And the answer to this question is implied in our previous investigations and will be fully developed in the last chapter. In the meantime we must never forget that the functional activity of this mind-body is mental, and can only be formulated in psychological terms. The concepts that we have used to explain conscious activity are all derived from psychological sources. The attempt to use physiological or physical ideas in explaining human or animal activity has everywhere broken down.

CHAPTER V

THE PSYCHOLOGY OF LANGUAGE

THE study of aphasia has shewn us that, as far as the psychology of language is concerned, no help is to be derived from investigations concerning the structure or function of the brain. Seeing that language is the most distinctively human function any account of human psychology which fails to deal with it is lopsided. Yet we find that, in so far as the topic is touched upon, we are treated to vague generalizations about universal language which probably never existed, or to detailed accounts of the structure of the vocal organs which are quite irrelevant, or to theories as to how language originated which the science of linguistics knows nothing about. The functioning of the vocal apparatus has about as much to do with the psychology of language as the instruments of an orchestra with appreciation of a symphony. Science does not deal with origins which lie beyond its ken. And although the grammarians of the early nineteenth century conceived of one original language from which all others were derived, this idea has now been abandoned by most philologists, although, as we shall see later, it has recently been suggested again on other grounds.

For a long time the idea was held that there existed somewhere or somehow a perfect language from which all languages were derived. An analagous thought occurs in the eleventh chapter of Genesis " And the whole earth was of one language and one speech . . . And the Lord said, Behold, they are one people, and they have all one language ; and this is what they begin to do : and now nothing will be withholden from them, which they purpose to do ". There was, it is thought, a time when the human spirit had complete control of its phonic material, a sort of golden age when the sounds chosen to express ideas were perfectly appropriate to them. As the material was, at that time, completely under the control of the creative spirit, thought was really able to embody itself in language. Then, like the Biblical Fall, there came a period of decadence ; and language was thenceforth submitted to the play of forces which corrupted and disorganized the work of the spirit. These forces worked independently of the human mind, and languages have gone on deteriorating in obedience to laws independent of volition. As we are now living in this decadent period we see around us the blind evolution of the various tongues and their consequent continual corruption. Purists in language and style constantly remind us of this.

There is one snare which the study of the psychology of language must avoid at all costs, namely the confusion between the epistemological and psychological standpoints. This may be illustrated by a quotation from Pick's *Die agrammatischen Sprachstörungen.* (1) He says " The act of formulating a schema of the sentence, and therefore the syntax and the corresponding part of the grammatical function, precedes the choice of words. The essential part of the psychical construction must be achieved from the grammatical point of view before the choice of words. We are compelled to admit that the psychological schema, that we have postulated on the analogy with the complex objective relations of the contents of thought, demands at first a grammatical scheme of the sentence corresponding to these relations. We may represent the development of this scheme, the representation of a whole which becomes effective by its decomposition into parts and is completed by words, by a schematic process of the grammatization of words ".

Thus we see that he distinguishes in an act of speech the following parts, the intuitive thought of what we are going to say, the mental formulation of this, the grammatical skeleton into which it is fitted, and finally the explicit verbal statement. Between the thought, or rather the attitude of mind or intention, and the expression in words, there are these series of intermediate stages. Now this is an excellent analysis of the epistemological structure of a sentence. But this well-ordered hierarchy of functions, founded on a complete analysis of what is implied in the ideal use of a language, has no place in a psychology of speech. It corresponds, in speech, to the syllogism or other logical schemes in reasoning, which may be implied in actual current reasoning, but are certainly not present to consciousness when a man argues.

For the most part we speak before having constructed the sentence ; we go immediately from the intention to the words. Thought is often analysed only at the moment of being expressed, the intermediate stages being skipped or greatly abbreviated, and more often only implied but never consciously formulated. Such rigorous analysis as is impiled in the above quotation is only possible at the end of a completed expression of thought—it is, as was said, epistemological not psychological, an ideal of a perfect logical language rather than a reality. It may be accomplished after the speaking is over by a logician, but is not present to the mind of the speaker, consciously or subconsciously, and therefore outside the purview of psychology.

It may help us to realize what does really happen in the evolution of a language if we start by inquiring how a child learns his mother-tongue ; for that is as near to origins as we are ever likely to get. The child has an inherited impulse to babbling, which is so strong and independent of all external impulsion that even the born deaf-mute babbles continually, so that his defects are not obvious at first. In addition, the human being is endowed with a strong tendency to imitate sounds and more especially human speech, being a kind of receiver attuned to such sounds. In this way the sounds which he spontaneously employs are enriched and extended ; and new sound combinations and rhythms are added to his babble repertoire. But a parrot can also imitate, and yet never acquires speech. There is added to the human endowment a third power, that of turning more or less spontaneously to an object when its name is mentioned. Without this, the most fundamental part of his innate capacity for language, true speech could never arise. In so far as any of the higher

animals possessed this power they would be on the road to
speech, but if they are entirely devoid of it, as seems probable,
there is an impassable chasm between the human and the
animal mind. When a dog learns to fetch an object in
response to a command or to turn to a person on hearing a
call this has nothing to do with language, but is a mere
association exactly similar to the association of smell with
food ; it is the so-called conditioned reflex. And even the
special barks indicative of hunger, delight, joy, etc., which
a dog indulges in are purely associative and devoid of thought
reference. A colour or sound which produces a conditioned
reflex in an animal is not the equivalent of a verbal sign ;
for as we shall see later a language is a system of relations,
and in reflex activity the relation is neither perceived nor
understood.

It is the development of this last faculty in its most
generalized form, the ability to realize that everything in
the universe has, or can have, a name that is the essence of
the faculty of language. Everything else is more or less
irrelevant, or merely a help to this fundamental capacity.
The child soon learns not only to turn to objects when their
name is mentioned but to perform simple acts which he is
spontaneously capable of, on being coaxed by words. Thus
he learns readily to clap his hands in response to a request,
and to perform other simple tasks which yield him delight.
There are thus, as Professor W. Stern (2) has pointed out,
three separate paths along which the child travels in order
to acquire his inheritance of speech ; active babble, imitation,
and the primitive understanding of the significance of names.
When these three paths unite he is well on the way to the
acquisition of his language inheritance.

It is quite impossible to understand the psychology of
language without drawing a sharp distinction between
associative and intelligent activity. A child may repeat a
sound, or a whole series of sounds, either spontaneously or
by association without using words. Thus he may babble
' mama ' for the mere love of the activity or even to betray
hunger ; but the babble sound only becomes a babble word

when he connects some independent meaning with it, *e.g.*
when he desires his mother or wishes to announce his hunger.
Unless, that is, the sound has some intended reference to
something outside itself, it is mere parrot-like association and
not a real word. In order to become a word the sound must
have some symbolic significance. A child may have been
babbling ' bow-wow ' by imitation for a long time till one
day he shows that he understands its significance by turning
to the dog. As soon as he is capable of using a symbol in this
way he does so with complete intelligence. It is not a question
of intelligence growing from a vaguer to a more complete
stage. The use of a symbol is a complete act of intelligence,
a flash of insight into a situation. Naturally, his intelligence
will grow with age, but as far as this particular act is concerned
it is as intelligent as it ever will be. With children who do
not learn to speak early, mimicry and gesture take the place
of sound language ; and gesture has the same symbolic
significance as the spoken word, but is more pictorial and
nearer to perceptual reality. In the use of speech and in
gesture the child can always understand much more than he
can spontaneously use, and this inferiority of the spoken
to the understood word remains all through life, for we all
of us possess a much smaller working vocabulary than the
reach of our understanding extends.

When children's babble becomes speech it displays characteristics of its own and is not merely a selection of words
from adult language. In a sense it employs more natural
sounds, seeing that onomatopoeic words and creations are
much more numerous and there are a considerable number
of sound expressing emotional states. Most children, if not
all, exhibit a tendency to invent words of their own for certain
objects and these nearly always have some sound resemblance
to the objects symbolized. Thus, a boy of about eighteen
months called all lights ' f.f.f.f.' which was really his imitation
of the sound of blowing out a light. As has been long recognized the first utterances of words are really sentences, and
consequently the same sound may have a variety of significa-
tions being helped out by cries, gestures and other movements.

It must also be remembered that a child's words have no very defined range of application. Having got hold of a word he will employ it for very diverse objects, provided only that there is some similarity, however vague, between such objects. The resemblance may reside not in the objects but in the child's reaction. Thus, for instance, a girl who was in the habit of pulling noses called all handles noses because she could pull them in the same way.

Students of phonetics and linguists have studied the so-called mutilations which language sounds undergo with time. They have in mind some standard or ideal forms from which the forms in daily use are thought to be deviations or corruptions. However that may be, and language apart from its use in intercourse seems to me an empty conception, we can trace in the language of early childhood all these deviations from an ideal norm. In this respect there is a parallelism between the development of the child and that of the race. Thus we find in children's speech substitution of dentals for gutturals (' dod ' for ' god ') assimilation of sounds (' gugar ' for ' sugar '), elisions (' ilk ' for ' milk '), metathesis (' waps ' for ' wasp '), condensations, displacements of sounds and so forth. It is interesting to observe that Freud in his dream interpretations finds similar substitutions, condensations and displacements in the imagery of dreams, which thus produce a distorted version of waking reality. This he attributes to some mythical censor who is guarding our thoughts, whereas the simple and obvious interpretation is that in dreaming we are dealing with a more primitive form of mentality, corresponding to that of childhood.

We called attention to the part played by imitation in the growth of speech, but it must be remembered that the human mind is never passive in any of its processes and that, therefore, imitation is never a gramophone reproduction of what is imitated. The child actively selects what he will imitate. From the flood of discourse which assails him on all sides he spontaneously, but of course, unintentionally, selects certain portions and in doing so he imitates certain persons in preference to others. And children spontaneously copy other children rather than adults. This process of selection is so remarkable that when more than one language is spoken in the presence of children they use now one and now another without mixing up the two. Since the main sounds, especially the consonants, are common to both languages it is patent that no explanation of this bi-lingual power in children is possible on the basis of brain localizations. Spontaneity and selectivity are so powerful that they may even over-ride the tendency to imitation. In the early stages of speech development, no matter how carefully the correct forms are uttered in a child's presence he prefers to use others which he creates, by analogy, from his existing store of forms. Thus he is fond of using ' ed ' to express the past tense and prefers ' goed ' to ' went ' and ' drinked ' to ' drunk ' no matter how often he hears the correct form. And if he is compelled to use the proper form, by correction, he still by analogy prefers to say ' wented ' to ' went '. This ability to employ analogy, often of a very remote kind, and the tendency to invent forms and phrases to express his language-hunger seems to me to remove the human mind from the sphere of natural selection.

Though the child, in his earliest language stages, tends to repeat in some manner the history of the race, yet the constraints imposed by his environment and the influence of adult speech soon eliminate this tendency. We may now inquire into the further stage of speech development beyond the primitive stage so far dealt with. Up till now we may say that speech has only been used on particular occasions to express isolated desires or emotions or to indicate pressing needs. But a tremendous step in advance is made when it is realized, for the first time, that everything in the world either has or can have a name. This is such an astounding discovery and the generalization is so vast that it may be regarded as a flash of intuitive genius. It is the child's first really general concept and instead of accepting it as a matter of course, we ought to be lost in admiration. And so indeed we should be, if we considered its implications, but since every child makes the discovery for himself we accept what is so common as a matter of course. Every parent is proud when a baby begins to walk or talk ; how much prouder ought he to be when his offspring shows himself capable of such an astonishing generalization. Imagine a dog or a chimpanzee capable of this feat !

By a stroke of luck we are able to be present at the moment when the blind deaf-mute Helen Keller (3) made this discovery for herself. She had learnt the names of several objects by having them spelt into her hand by means of the manual alphabet. This was a purely associative connection such as an animal makes ; and in this way she had learnt about thirty words regarding them purely as a game. She found great difficulty in learning the verb ' to drink ' and confused it with the words ' mug ' and ' milk ' ; going through the pantomime of drinking whenever the latter words were spelled. Her teacher noted the day when it flashed upon her that everything has a name, and that the manual alphabet was the key to everything she wanted to know. It happened in this way. " It occurred to me that with the help of this new word [water] I might succeed in straightening out the ' mug-milk ' difficulty. We went into the pump house, and I made Helen hold her mug under the spout while I pumped. As the cold water gushed forth, filling the mug, I spelled w-a-t-e-r into Helen's free hand. The word coming so close upon the sensation of cold water rushing over her hand seemed to startle her. She dropped the mug and stood as one trans-fixed. A new light came into her face. She spelled ' water ' several times. Then she dropped on the ground and asked for its name and pointed to the pump and the trellis, and suddenly turning round she asked for my name. . . . All the way back to the house she was highly excited, and learned the name of every object she touched, so that in a few hours she had added thirty new words to her vocabulary."

This insight into the symbolic significance of words is, as we have said, something very different from a mere perceptual or associative process. Advance is now very rapid and the child's vocabulary is greatly enlarged, so that at the age of two to two-and-a-half a normal child has a vocabulary of 300 words. The dominance of the one-word sentence begins to give way, and words are now connected into phrases. At first interjection sentences, expressing emotion or will, as opposed to statements are in the ascendant. The child's first sentences are disjointed in structure, like telegrams ; and the order of words is very expressive since the important words come at the beginning or the end, depending on the momentary mood of the child. It is only very gradually and by dint of much practice that the usual order of words is acquired and inflexions are correctly used. Conjunctions, relative pronouns, etc., are slow in coming and their meaning is given largely by intonation. The purely childish stage of speech ends when he is capable of constructing subordinate sentences at the approximate age of four or five. There are other stages, of course, but these later developments are of incomparably less importance psychologically than the stages we have traced.

All through these early stages and especially the last, the spontaneity of the child is exhibited by the creation of new word forms to fill up gaps in his vocabulary. This evinces a strong natural feeling for language and makes the assumption that learning is merely the establishment of a series of conditioned reflexes appear preposterous. A conditioned reflex or any other form of physiological process can never be creative, but there are numerous instances where children invent a language for use amongst themselves ; sometimes, but not always, founded on adult language. The influence of subjective selection is shewn in the relative numbers of the different parts of speech which occur in a child's vocabulary. As compared with an adult a child uses relatively more verbs, *i.e.* words expressive of action, and relatively less adjectives. Thus it has been estimated that an adult's vocabulary contains eleven per cent. of verbs and twenty-two per cent of adjectives ; whereas a child of three years employs only five per cent of adjectives but twenty per cent of verbs. (4)

It is now time to turn from the acquirement of language by children to the question of the psychology of language in general ; only there is no language in general, there are only languages. It is most unfortunate that writing was ever invented, or grammar discovered, for both of these confuse the psychology of language. The ideal language for our purpose would be one which had never been reduced to writing. The written word exercises a tyrannical influence over the spoken word in literary languages, owing to the prestige of the writers. Whilst the spoken language goes on evolving the written word remains comparatively fixed. But writing is a mere attempt at a photographic reproduction of spoken language and quite external to it. The most original treatment of the subject is that given by F. de Saussure in a work called *Cours de Linguistique générale.* (5) He points out that language is both a product of evolution and a social institution and works out both these ideas in a highly suggestive manner. We must distinguish carefully between what is inborn in a language from that which is conventional. At first sight it might appear that our vocal apparatus is made for speaking, much as our legs are intended for walking. But gestures could equally well have been employed, or some other visual forms, as in the manual language of the dumb, or even tactile motor impressions as with blind deaf-mutes. In the latter case the ' speech centre ' in the brain would have to be located in the motor area of the cortex. What is natural to man is the faculty prompting him to employ a set of signs to denote ideas and objects, or the power of symbolization. The process of symbolic thinking however, must not be considered as a mere juxtaposition of a symbol and an idea, much as a label is stuck on an object. The unity of signifier and signified is a very special and intimate one ; a solidarity with two aspects. Combined with this there is the innate tendency to give expression to our emotional states by cries or gestures, or some other variety of movement. We shall deal first with the contribution of emotion to language.

Sir Richard Paget (6) has propounded a theory of the origin of speech according to which gesture and the movements of articulation are the important elements, and phonation is simply an accident. " It is to the movements of articulation that we must go—not to the intangible sounds—if we would discover the riddle of human speech." He believes that there

H

is an inborn association between the movements of a man's hands and mouth. The original form of expression of a man's ideas was bodily pantomime and the mouth and tongue movements unconsciously copied these. Every bodily gesture was accompanied by a sympathetic mouth gesture, and when a man desired to make others attend to him he made an unconscious emotional cry by forcing air through the mouth. In course of time the hand gestures fell into abeyance as the hand was required for other purposes ; and only the mouth gesture and the ensuing phonation were much in evidence. The particular sounds that would result are entirely accidental and determined by the shape of the mouth cavity resulting from the tongue and lip gestures. In some such way as this Paget thinks that all primitive roots of words have a natural gesture meaning which a clever anatomist and phonetician could decipher. And it would seem to follow that all languages must have common roots which have been disguised and corrupted by usage. In this sense there might have been a time when the whole earth was of one language and one speech as conceived in the story in Genesis. Whilst, however, philologists deny the common origin of the roots of all languages, the insistence on emotional expression as one of the fundamental bases of speech gives the theory a certain psychological validity.

The importance of emotional expression as one of the roots of language has long been recognized. There are for example some aboriginal races who cannot carry on a discussion in the dark ; they must light a fire to see one another's gestures and facial expression. But what is sometimes overlooked is the fact that emotional expression cannot become language unless it is in some way symbolized. Emotions are expressed in some form of movement which renders them visible to others. But with children such movements are inchoate and involve the whole body. Gradually they become more restricted and definite, and so more expressive. At the highest stages of language development the emotions may be expressed by differences of intensity, pitch and timbre in speech, accompanied by gestures, so that a good actor can simulate very delicate shades of feeling. Yet, as some emotions are too intimate to be communicable, part of our affective life remains inexpressible. For there are deep emotions so profound as to prevent us from symbolizing them; and others so vague and fleeting as to be too subtle to grasp in language even by the great masters of language, the poets. In ordinary conversation our affective life is expressed, not by words, but by gestures, inflexions, intonation, rhythm, etc. As Professor H. Delacroix has so well expressed it : " Donner le ton juste avec ses intensités, ses assourdissments, l'allongement, l'élevation des syllabes et des mots, mettre l'accent, s'arrêter, ralentir, accélérer, faire ressortir ou escamoter, telle est l'oeuvre du sentiment ."

When our spontaneous cries and mimicry are seen to serve their purpose we repeat them for the purposes of communication. Thus a child first cries because he feels pain ; and when he perceives that this is understood he thereafter uses such cries to summon others to his aid. What was originally a mere expression of feeling becomes in this way a sign ; and in a similar manner gestures and other involuntary movements become conventional symbols. We employ them to express what we wish to express after having previously used them to express what we were unable to express.

To propound the psychology of language would be to write the history of social groups. For language is above all else a social product. It is by means of this institution which society has created that the individual is able to exercise his inborn language faculty, his tendency to employ symbols. The constraints of society model the habits of its members and so breed common habits of thought and speech. Individual experience is thus both dominated and sustained by the traditional institution of speech. But we must always remember that a society of individuals could never produce anything unless individuals themselves were creative ; so that the growth of language assumes that changes are introduced by individuals and adopted by society. We are apt to think of institutions as something material, overlooking the fact that what gives them form and significance are the ideas and aspirations implied in them, which the material forms merely help to perpetuate. In the same way a language is a purely psychical entity existing independently of individuals and yet embodied in them, just as the reality of a symphony is independent of the particular manner of its execution. On the other hand there is something entirely individual about the word as opposed to the language of which it is part. For a word is a psycho-physical existent ; something uttered or heard, or in some other way expressed. It exists only momentarily. No doubt a word and a language both imply each other, for a language is necessary in order that the word may be intelligible and words are essential in order that a language may embody itself.

In considering the psychological function of words it is essential to confine ourselves to oral words and ignore other modes of communication. Now an oral word implies a hearer, even if the hearer should be the speaker himself. The acoustic image is intimately united with the act of phonation so as to constitute a unity. But a word obviously implies some concept, without which it would have no significance whatever. We may call the acoustic image (together with the phonation) the signifier, and the concept the signified ; though it must be admitted that these names are awkward. It will be observed that both the signifier and the signified are psychical. When we say that a word is a sign or a symbol it is necessary to bear in mind that the sign has this double nature. If either aspect is omitted the other is a mere psychological abstraction. A spoken chain of sounds no matter how they are connected is simply a physiological phenomenon entirely devoid of psychological meaning. As we have seen it is impossible to understand the phenomena of aphasia on a physiological basis. The symbolic signification of language resides in this bond of union between the two psychical elements, whereby reference is made to something external to both of them. Images have no signification apart from the concepts and these latter could get no purchase on the world without the former. The bond of union between the two, which constitutes a sign, is entirely arbitrary except in the rare case of onomatopoeic words. And this sign of course, always refers to something which is neither the image nor the concept. It is such external reference which makes it a symbol.

Difficulties frequently arise in psychological discussions from the confusion between a mental image and a concept. What distinguishes the two is the fact that a concept unlike an image, holds in solution a number of judgments. Such judgments are gradually crystallized out as thinking becomes more definite and speech develops. The latent judgments always assume relations between concepts, so that there is a sense in which it is true to say that any concept virtually involves all others. When an idea arises all other ideas exist potentially in the mind. Plato's doctrine of reminiscence whereby all that a man is destined to know he has already known but forgotten is simply an inverted way of expressing this truth. Owing to the close relation between thought and language it follows that when a word is formulated a whole language exists in potentiality. We must also bear in mind that an image, with its associated concept, only has a symbolic significance because it is not taken for what it appears but for what it suggests. It is this representative function which is the essence of a system of signs or symbols.

We thus see that the fundamental part of the language faculty is the power to understand and employ signs or symbols. The written word, as we have indicated, is a bar to understanding the psychological significance of language. For much of the value of words resides in difference of intonation and the associative context in the mind of the speaker or listener. The universe of discourse which words inhabit is responsible for their meaning. Even the earliest words of a child, as we have seen, are sentences ; and an isolated word is a mere abstraction, having no independent existence except in the pages of a dictionary. All the difficulties arising from the physiological view of aphasia may be referred to the misconception that words have an existence apart from a context. If a foreigner only knew the meaning of the word ' love ' from a dictionary how could he understand the following passage from a letter of the poet Cowper to his cousin Harriet :

" So much as I love you I wonder how the deuce it has happened that I was never in love with you ".

When a person speaks he produces, as it were, a ribbon of sound. In early Hebrew manuscripts the words are written without spaces between them and the sentences are not divided from each other. This is an excellent pictorial representation of spoken language, except that to represent it more accurately all the letters should run into one another or be continuous. In listening to an unknown language there is no method by which we can cut up the ribbon of sound so as to distinguish the separate words. Perhaps it may be thought that this difficulty would not occur with one's own language, and that a sensitive ear could pick out the separate words. But this a pure blunder.

There has been a controversy as to whether English poetry consisted of ' quantity ' verse in which long and short syllables occur, or ' stress verse ', composed of strong and weak syllables. Mr E. W. Scripture (7) submitted spoken verse to experimental investigation to decide this point. A person speaks into a tube and the movements of the air are recorded on a paper by a light lever attached to a membrane ; whilst a tuning fork records the time. It is found that the record of speech thus obtained is without breaks. It does not resemble *in any way* the printed text, nor does the record give any indication of what the ear is supposed to hear. " Anybody with a prejudice can be made to hear anything ; all that is needed is to create the proper expectation ". What gives verse its distinctive quality is a combination of four elements, quality of enunciation, loudness, duration of vowels or consonants or combinations of these, and differences of pitch. Long syllables are often louder, more precisely enunciated and higher in pitch, so that what we call length may be due to melody, whilst the records do not shew that long syllables are actually longer as regards time of utterance. Except where pauses are deliberately made speech is a course of continuous action, not a series of disconnected words. Just as the foot strikes the floor at regular intervals in dancing, but these strokes are only phases in a continuous movement, so speech is a smooth flow of sound. Graphic records obtained, in the way indicated, shew not the faintest trace of any division into words nor, it may be added, of verse into feet. Still less do the single letters stand out within a word. In fact it has been strongly maintained that metric systems are purely artificial systems of treating printed verse and have no counterpart at all in real speech.

It is evident from what has now been said that if we are to understand the psychology of language the study of words is misleading. For the same phonetic section of sound may, by differences of context, express very different ideas. This is true even when there are no differences of intonation or emphasis to mark the distinction, as when we speak of ' adopting a fashion ' or ' adopting a child '. In fact the identity of a word in speech, as opposed to that of the printed word which is an artificial identity, exactly corresponds to those other identities where the material is unimportant but the sameness is psychical. We speak of the same street, though from one generation to another all the houses may have been completely reconstructed from new material and the road completely changed. Similarly, we refer to the same train though all the rolling stock has changed and the engines are of a new type. In all these cases the identity is obviously not material but is founded on certain conditions to which the accidental matter happens to conform. The identity is real enough and has a material embodiment but is in no sense itself a material identity. Linguistic identity has a similar meaning, being founded not on the same material but on certain psychological conditions. These considerations, by themselves, if we had no other evidence, would be sufficient to render absurd the idea that word images are somehow stored in the brain. For since the identity of a word with prior examples of itself is an identity of conditions we have no use for permanent images to safeguard the identity.

This idea may perhaps be rendered a little clearer if we compare the words of a language to the pieces in a game of chess, though it must be admitted that the analogy is very rough. A particular piece of wood or ivory may have a certain form and we call it a Knight or a Queen. But should it be lost or broken any other object may be used in its place and the game in no way suffers. What makes a Knight or Queen is obviously not a particular shape or material but a certain assigned value. Such value makes any Knight identical with any other. Should Capablanca's suggestion be adopted of a board with a hundred squares and new pieces, the values of all the pieces will automatically change. It must further be remarked that the effective value of all the pieces is changing all through the game. And, whereas, in chess the values may perhaps be regarded as static at any moment of the game, in a language the values are always dynamic. When we are considering the psychology of language the notion of identity is closely bound up with the idea of value.

To this notion of linguistic value we must now devote some attention. A child learning to speak or a man learning a new language is engaged in acquiring a system of values. For this reason schoolmasters have learnt that the only effective way of learning a foreign language is to employ the ' direct ' method. However well the grammar is known or the vocabulary extended the language is never learnt, but is always artificial, until we feel our way into its values by using it in the same way that the linguistic group does.

Language is, then, a system of pure values embodied in a system of purely arbitrary signs. Economists distinguish between exchange value and utility value ; and the same aspects of value can be found in language. Thus a chair has a value to a manufacturer because he can exchange it for cash, that is, its value is determined by dissimilar things ; whereas it has a different sort of value to the purchaser who compares it, for his purpose, to other chairs or sofas, that is to similar things. Similarly words possess a value in that they can be, as it were, exchanged for ideas ; but they can also be compared with other words. We may call the former value their significance and the latter their linguistic value ; and it is obviously impossible to separate these, though we may analytically consider them apart. The above distinction can perhaps be better realized by means of an example. The

French word *mouton* has the same significance as the English
sheep since the same idea is involved, and each is the sign of
the same objective reality, a particular species of animal.
Nevertheless the words have not the same linguistic value,
since the Englishman does not ask for sheep at the dinner
table but for mutton. As the word sheep has another word
with which it may be compared whilst the word mouton has
not, there is a difference in the linguistic value. Within any
one language the words which express synonymous ideas
limit one another's application, for if the synonymous words
did not exist all the significance would reside in one and the
same word. In a somewhat similar fashion all the words in
a sentence limit or enrich the rest, and it is evident that
linguistic values are almost entirely a matter of context.
And further, it is the linguistic system as a whole which
influences the values of all the expressions in it.

What has been said about words is equally true of the
grammatical system of a language. The value of a plural in
English is not equivalent to that in Greek or Hebrew since
these latter have a dual form which expresses part of the
value of an English plural ; and Fijian has a dual, a trial,
and a plural. Again, distinctions of tense in grammar as
representing time relationships do not exist in Hebrew. The
verb has two forms signifying completed or uncompleted
actions. With these forms distinctions of time can be represented from any particular standpoint. So we see that, what
might have been regarded as an essential feature of language,
if we confined ourselves to Indo-European tongues, is but an
accidental point of view. It is evident that the point of view
in these languages is somewhat different from that in English.
Thought, like spoken language, is originally an amorphous
mass in which certain divisions are made to correspond to
separate ideas. These separate parts are sometimes, but by
no means always, provided with linguistic signs to enable us
to make ourselves intelligible to ourselves and to others.
The stream of thought and the phonic stream are both split
up into corresponding systems, so that the ideas signified
and the system of signifiers more or less correspond. It is

doubtful whether systematic thinking could go on, and it is certain that it could not go far, without the corresponding signs. For without them it would be nebulous or hazy. This is the element of truth in the controversy which raged in the nineteenth century as to whether language was necessary for thought.

Both ideas and the phonetic material in which they are expressed thus constitute systems and it is this which gives them their psychological values. Such values, as we have seen, being purely relational can be modified by modifying the context. This is true of each system taken separately. But a linguistic system implies both series intimately fused into one ; and such unity engenders a new system of values different from either. This latter system constitutes the effective bond between each signifier and what is signified. Though the signified and the signifiers, each taken by themselves have a purely relational value, their combination into a unified system yields values which are concrete and, more or less, self-sustaining. It is this linguistic system of values as a whole, existing in a person or rather in a group of persons, which resists change and gives a language a certain measure of stability. Whatever language we examine we find this constitutive feature, a complex system of values in equilibrium in which the parts condition one another. F. de Saussure to whom we owe this conception of language as a system of values expresses the idea thus : " La langue est une forme et non une substance ". By this Aristotelian *dictum* he desired to call attention to the fact that the values in a language are just as immaterial as the values in a work of art.

For purposes of exposition it has been necessary to consider the relational values of a language as though thought was purely linear. Since the words of a sentence must be uttered in time, or written one after another, the chain of words unrolls itself in a linear fashion. Each word, as it comes, has relations with the rest, and the corresponding values arising from such a linear relationship. But words have other relationships and consequently other values. Just as we can speak of the thread of thought so we can, in a more appropriate metaphor, consider the fabric of our thinking, in which the threads form the warp and the woof. Each word is the centre not only of a linear series but has associative relations with a wide range of other terms, which are not necessarily present in consciousness when a sentence is uttered. This large array of potential associates, present subconsciously when a word it uttered, is responsible for a further set of values in which the word is enshrined. So that the full meaning of a sentence is largely potential rather than actual, and the associative connections being different in different people give a different colouring to the whole. Such associative relationships breed a new set of values peculiar to each person.

It was said previously that a language was a social institution, but up to the present we have confined our attention mainly to its development in individuals. It is desirable at this point to emphasize the social aspect. For any language is the common work of a linguistic group, who impose it on successive generations. Each language as has been aptly said, is a historical variation on the great human theme of language. We have seen that a language is a system whose parts interpenetrate and maintain each other by their solidarity. Such a strongly organized system of values, pre-existent as far as any individual is concerned, impresses itself on the thought of each one, and like other stable institutions can only be modified by a process of slow evolution. The evolution of a language as a social institution is to a certain extent fortuitous. Its complexity and arbitrary character resists change, since there is no better defence against reasonable change than to be unreasonable.

As regards the complex character we have to consider not a single but a triple evolution. For a language consists, as has been previously shewn, of a phonetic system or the phonic material, a vocabulary in which this material gets definite form, and a morphological system comprising the grammar. Each of these has separate characteristics, and modification may ensue from any of them. It is by ignoring this extreme complexity and considering language as a single system that innumerable difficulties about the psychology of language and the nature of aphasia have arisen. A word is a totality of functions, combined in the effort to communicate, by which a person speaking utilizes the institution of language to express his personal thought. Theories of aphasia which regard words as simple phonic or acoustic objects and overlook the fact that words are combinations of sound, sense and grammatical relationships are bound to be futile. And the hypothesis of cerebral localization is a striking example of the error due to over simplification.

As regards the arbitrary and illogical character of language this is doubtless true of the great majority of speakers, who perpetuate routine by blindly following tradition. Yet as Mons. A. Sechehaye (8) points out, there are artists and geniuses in language who impose their views on a whole people and in this way determine what form the system shall take. Language does not, therefore, express the spontaneous individuality of the person speaking and is not subject to every passing whim. The ordinary person expresses his thought and feeling in ways determined for him by artists in language, who are the persons who make the tradition. Ordinary people find a system ready made and submit to it. This tradition however, by its resistance to spontaneous arbitrary changes, enables the ordinary speaker to express himself more accurately, and to feel more finely, than he would do if he had to create expressions for himself. Artist's creations become part of the linguistic system of values and general convention enables them to survive. It is only by following the beaten track, and utilizing the landmarks already made, that the average individual is able to express himself freely and to utilize logical and other distinctions that he would be powerless to make for himself. In so far as a Shakespeare or a Dante is responsible for the evolution of a language it ceases to be entirely arbitrary. Nevertheless, for the majority of speakers in the world at large, it is no doubt true that the evolution is the result of a multitude of arbitrary and illogical causes.

There is a prevailing idea of long standing that a language in some way expresses the soul of a people, and, as a conse quence, that we may by examining the language infer the inherited characteristics of a race. But if this is intended to mean that a particular tongue is a racial attribute much as the shape of the skull or the colour of the skin it is a blunder. The Greek word idiom (idioma = a special custom) gets nearer to the correct view, for a language is a habit not a racial peculiarity. Diversity of race is no bar to the existence amongst a nation of a common tongue. The causes which determine the spread of a language are sociological, political, etc., and not primarily psychological. Unity of race is only a secondary factor in determining what a national language shall be. And it is to social, political or religious unity that we must look to find the causes that establish a linguistic community. Conversely, linguistic unity is one of the most powerful factors in creating a nation out of diverse racial groups, as we see exemplified in the melting pot of the United States of America.

It is very dangerous to infer the mentality of a people from their language, either its vocabulary or its structure. No doubt the genius of a people tends to preserve certain forms or words once they have been adopted, but there is hardly a characteristic of any language which cannot be paralleled in others, however wide apart. As Mr A. M. Hocart (9) has pointed out, as a result of his study of the South Sea islanders, many things which appear strange to us in their languages have exact parallels in our own. Thus the Fijians have different possessive pronouns in such phrases as ' my coat ' and ' my bread '. But does this mean that they are less capable of discerning identity in difference or of generalizing ? Not at all ; for we have exactly this peculiarity since we have words for a bull, a cow, an ox, a calf, etc., but none for the species except ' cattle ' or ' kine ' which are collective terms. Again the South Sea islanders have nine different names for the coconut at different stages of its growth ; but it would be a mistake to attribute this to the richness of their language or power of discernment, since it is merely an expression of the fact that at each stage it has for them some practical utility. Englishmen who reside in those parts adopt some of these terms for such as are of practical use to them. These same islanders have different words for different operations which we do not distinguish, such as cutting a yam lengthwise or crosswise ; but then there is a vital difference in these processes for planting. In a similar fashion Mr Bertram Thomas the explorer has pointed out that if you ask an inhabitant of Southern Arabia to describe a particular land he will inevitably refer to its water supply. But who could fail to do this in such a climate ?

The fact that a language is primitive, though it would be hard to define what is meant by primitive in this connection, is no more an indication of a low mental development than the use of stone implements where iron has never been thought of. A primitive man might with apparent justice accuse us of having more words than ideas and point to such examples as end, finish ; begin, commence ; god, deity, etc. Of course it is not possible to understand these redundant words without a knowledge of the history of the nation ; and similar peculiarities or deficiencies in primitive peoples may also be due to historical causes, mixtures of peoples and so on. We are too apt to build theories of mental development on the peculiarities of vocabulary among primitive peoples, forgetting that those who are not interested in certain things do not require words for those things. Thus, as Mr Hocart says : " What a European, continually using a savage language, wearies of is not the excess of minute distinctions, but the vagueness of concepts so wide that they cannot convey the distinctions which he takes an interest in and which alone makes conversation worth while to him ; he cannot speak of trees without including all plants ; he cannot take the birds and leave the bats and butterflies ; he has but one word to use whether he is discussing ambition, rivalry or jealousy ; in translating *lialia* into English he must consider whether mad, foolish, simple, idiotic or ignorant will suit the context because English has no word to express intellectual deficiency in general. . . . The language seems so poor to him simply because he insists on saying things that *he* takes a detailed interest in, but not the Fijian. . . . Let him turn to planting, to handicrafts, and war, and he will find as precise and minute a vocabulary as he may require ".

If we now attempt to sum up the contribution that our study of the psychology of language has made to the mind-body problem, we shall be helped by an analogy. The material system of a language consists of the phonic material that is employed, out of which the vocabulary is constructed ; and the grammar may be considered as the analogue of the morphology of organic bodies. Just as material bodies have their own laws of development so the sonorous material obeys certain phonetic laws. As soon, however, as we try to formulate what these laws are we see that it is not possible to do so without reference to the mind of the person speaking. Phonic material is animated by psychical laws, without which there is nothing but sound and fury, signifying nothing. There is no doubt, of course, that pronunciation may change independently of all consideration of sense or grammar, and the best known of such changes are formulated in Grimm's law. But such modifications concern only the artificially isolated elements of sounds within words and, as such, have little to do with language proper. What these changes are due to has led to much speculation, but they are most probably the result of social habit. It has been supposed that certain races have a tendency to produce diverse sounds, but there is no reason whatever to suppose the vocal apparatus varies with race. A group of German babies brought up in England by English mothers would have their foster mother's pronunciation. For the same differences of pronunciation are apparent in smaller local groups within a linguistic unity as differences of dialect or accent. But a determined effort and education can change such local variations, as we see in the changes of accent as the result of easier intercourse between the different parts of a country.

It has been thought that phonetic changes may be explained by the law of economy of effort, *i.e.* that more difficult articulations give way to easier. No doubt this does occur within any linguistic group but it is hard to understand why one nation should prefer more difficult articulation ; and moreover it is impossible to say what is more or less easy to pronounce. It is all a matter of custom and habit. What habit has stamped into a person's speech a determined and prolonged effort can eradicate. And although the process of phonation becomes almost unconscious, so that we speak without being aware of the movements of articulation, yet it never becomes purely reflex. For, when we speak, the whole process is subject to the guiding force of what we wish to say, and it is under the dominion of this dominant idea that the phrases are unfolded. In moments of absent mindedness, when conscious control is temporarily lost, we utter phrases we did not intend, but we are promptly made aware of them, shewing that the process is never completely unconscious. Normally however, our discourse is guided by the prevailing intention. So that a separation between what is material and what is psychical in speech is artificial. Just as a living organism is a mind-body in which the guiding forces are psychical so a language is a unity in which the material part is completely under the directing control of the spiritual. It requires a mind with definite ideas to convert the chaotic babble of sound which the vocal apparatus is capable of producing into a linguistic system. As far as the individual is concerned he is helped to the acquisition of this system by virtue of his membership of a social group in which the system is strongly entrenched.

Professor H. Delacroix (10) who has dealt with the psychology of language in his admirable work *Le Langage et la pensée* thus describes what a child has to do in acquiring language values in his mother tongue. " L'attitude mentale de l'enfant qui comprend et qui parle doit donc s'élargir jusqu'à la mesure de cet univers logique et verbal. Analyser la continuité sonore du discours entendu, décomposer la phrase, des flexions, déduire les relations logiques, retenir dans une appréhension simultanée cette mélodie évancescente et qui se construit à mesure qu'elle s'évanouit, construire au fur et à mesure un ensemble sur des éléments qui disparaissent au fur et à mesure, faire une synthèse en même temps qu'une analyse, aller de l'intelligence de l'ensemble à l'intelligence des éléments et *vice versa*, tel est le jeu d'opérations fort complexes qu'à partir d'un certain degré et sous une certaine forme la comprehension du langage met inévitablement en oeuvre ". This summary expresses but part of what any language involves ; and makes it preposterous to suppose that any activity short of a creative and regulative intelligence has been at work, and is perpetually at work, in forming the system of values which constitute a language.

Thus we realize that verbal symbols are not merely sounds taking the place of things. A system of words is only a language when the mind is capable of perceiving in their succession a simultaneous unity which itself has constructed. It is the essence of symbols to break with the things they represent ; to construct a network of relations, to effect operations on the relations of the things signified and to justify assertions about such relations. All such operations, though controlled by objective reality, are operations by thought on thought.

I

Chapter VI

THE PSYCHOLOGY OF TEMPERAMENT

Ever since classical times there has persisted a belief in a direct relation of the body to the mind, the temperamental relation, according to which the mind is a reflection of the constitution of the body. This doctrine arose in a peculiar way and is an illuminating example of the persistence of psychological error resulting from discarded physiological beliefs. The Greeks believed that the universe was composed of two pairs of opposites, namely the hot and the cold, the moist and the dry. These opposites were the essential qualities of the four elements, fire, air, water and earth. Empedocles thought that these elements were also the components of the human body, and that disease was due to an excess of one or the other of them. The most famous physician of antiquity, Hippocrates (460–377 B.C.) (1), taught, however, that the body was composed of four humours and that health consisted in a harmonious blending of these. There is some doubt as to what these humours were, but usually they were enumerated as blood, phlegm, yellow and black bile; though in the writings of Hippocrates the first two are the most prominent, whilst other authors included a watery humour instead of one of the biles. Half a millenium after Hippocrates the other classical physician Galen, though he disagreed with the philosophical basis of the former, believed strongly in the doctrine of temperaments. He wrote " Those who think that the soul is not helped or hindered by the temperament of the body have nothing to say of the differences between children and can give no reason for the diversity which makes some bold and others cowardly, or some intelligent and others stupid." (2) This is the doctrine of temperament in a nutshell.

Amid all differences that arose there was agreement on

one common principle, that health is a harmonious mingling of these constituents, whatever they are. Nobody was quite clear as to what was to be meant by ' harmonious ' or what was implied in ' mingling ', but this did nothing to prevent the doctrine from spreading over the civilized world. As there were four elements and four humours in the body, there must be four temperaments ; for the mind is a reflection from the body. And to this day we have the sanguine, the bilious, the melancholic and the phlegmatic, each corresponding to one of the classical humours. The difficulty of shaking off this number four is shewn by the fact that Kant, who held the Greek view, derived the number, not from the elements, but from the syllogism. As this had four figures there could be four temperaments only, not any other number. Richerand, an eighteenth century physiologist, added a fifth, the nervous temperament ; and this was a distinct advance. For, by the introduction of the nervous system the functional view of temperament was emphasized. He meant by a nervous temperament the sensibility to impressions on our organs, which could be weak or strong. Though I have called this a fifth class, it would perhaps be better to say that it was a qualification of the other four, since he describes sensibility to impressions as varying with the sanguine, the bilious and so on. (2)

An ingenious recent attempt has been made to derive the four temperaments from two main roots, depending on a person's powers of inhibition. Some people seem to lack this power and react with unusual vigour to any situation. Such are the hyperkinetic, who are characterized by exaltation, irritability or psycho-motor excitement. The extreme examples are very violent and threatening, and in pathological cases this lack of inhibition may develop into the manic—depressive psychosis. Ordinarily, however, such people are braggarts, conceited, hyper-erotic and suffer from violent fits of destructiveness or temper. Of this temperament there are two grades, the lesser being the nervous and the more developed the choleric. Opposed to these we have the hypokinetic, who are over inhibited. They respond with difficulty to any situation. Their thoughts and actions are retarded and their emotions deep and stable. They are apt to worry over trifles, to brood and to suffer from anxiety. In extreme cases they feel life a burden too hard to endure. Of this sort there are also two grades, the lesser inhibited are the phlegmatic, and the greater the melancholic. (3)

No important change in the conception of the physiological doctrine of the temperaments has been made for two thousand years, except that the emphasis has shifted from the constituents of the body to their functioning, and that different constituents have been evoked. From the time that the study of the nervous system began to be pursued there has emerged a tendency to consider temperaments as being due to its tone or function rather than to its structure. But with the discovery of the ductless glands there has once again arisen a belief that the humours, which are now called hormones, are responsible for the variety of temperaments. There are round about half-a-dozen endocrine glands, so that there ought to be this number of temperaments, but the number four is too firmly fixed to be so easily dislodged, except in favour of the number two corresponding to the Greek opposites. Besides, the number of endocrine glands may be increased by future research, unlike the four Greek elements which were eternal and immutable.

According, then, to the view which we have inherited from the past and have re-adapted to meet modern physiology, temperament is a part of man's innate constitution ; the effect of his bodily organs on his character. The fund of tendencies which express his emotional mode of reacting, the tone of his organs, the general direction of his vitality ; all of these are nowadays said to be determined by the hormones secreted by his endocrine glands ; and these are his temperament. This doctrine reached its culminating point when Dr L. Berman wrote a book with the title, *Glands regulating Personality.* According to him the " Chemistry of the cell is the chemistry of the soul ", whatever that may mean. We are, in fact, gland controlled marionettes. Just as a dose of alcohol may make a man happy, or a dose of cocaine make him feel that there are no obstacles in the world, so doses of internal secretion may determine his temperament and thereby his personality. Dr Berman (4) informs us that " the grey matter of the brain, the glands of internal secretion, the pituitaries, the pineal, the thymus, the thyroid and the parathyroids, the liver and the pancreas, the adrenals and the sex glands, constitute the core of our personality, because they are the mediators between the individual and the environment. There is nothing in an environment to which they are not sensitive and responsive." Now this is a bit unfair, for the nervous system and the digestive organs are smuggled in to help out the endocrine glands in regulating our personality. The functions of the nervous system have already been fully dealt with in earlier chapters. What we are now interested in is the theory that our temperaments depend on the hormones secreted by the internal glands.

The thyroid and the adrenal glands are the two about which our knowledge is most definite. Thyroid deficiency leads to stunted growth and may produce melancholia, and the complete absence of the gland is accompanied by idiocy or mental deficiency. The general mental depression which results from lack of functioning of the thyroid, and the stunted growth may be relieved by thyroid extract. It is believed that. the function of the thyroid hormone is to handle the iodine which enters the body as food, producing a compound which regulates the level of energy production in the cells of the body. As to the adrenals, their hormone serves to stimulate the liver to discharge its sugar, which again is an energizing substance necessary for muscular activity. So that the purpose of the two chief endocrine glands is to regulate, not personality but the chemical energy of the body. It does not add very much to our psychological knowledge to learn that in order to face the world efficiently our bodies must somehow be provided with the means of energizing the food we take in ; and this would seem to be the main function of the ductless glands. More to the purpose is the function of the sex-organs, acting as endocrine glands. It is said that femininity depends on the elaboration of substance secreted by the ovaries, and that in this way adolescence and other changes may be explained. Similar influence is said to be exerted in men by the secretions of the prostate. But all these organs have been shewn to do is to stimulate the full growth of certain secondary or sex linked characters.

Certain drugs, such as alcohol, morphine, or cocaine, influence psychic events in one of two ways, either by exciting or depressing our general affective tone or changing the psychic tempo. On this basis Professor McDougall (5) builds an ingenious argument to shew how the endocrine glands are the regulators of temperament. " If a man possessed an organ whose metabolism generated alcohol he would, whenever this organ was stirred to increased activity, exhibit a change of temperament of the nature of alcoholic intoxication ; for drunkenness in its milder degrees is nothing but a temporary modification of temperament through the influence of alcohol on the processes of the brain. It is probable that every tissue of the body contributes to determine temperament in this chemical fashion. But certain tissues are of vastly greater influence than others. Chief amongst these are the ductless glands." This attractive theory loses a good deal of its force when the mental effects of alcohol and similar substances are taken into account. Alcohol has a sedative effect, and therefore removes emotional inhibitions ; but if it is taken constantly this effect passes off and the dose has to be increased. The danger of alcohol and other drugs lies just in this, that frequent use necessitates an increase in amount to get any mental effect at all. It must be remembered that adrenalin and secretions of the other endocrine glands are produced in very minute quantities, necessitating delicate chemical tests for their detection. If, then, they produced any mental effect this would long since have worn off and the glands would have to produce constantly increasing quantities. Their physiological effects are no doubt very pronounced and important, but it would be as reasonable to expect us to taste the saliva which is constantly moistening the mouth as to suppose that hormones can effect our conscious experience.

There is, in addition, physiological evidence which negatives the supposition that temperament is determined by glandular

activity.   Professor W. B. Cannon (6) studied experimentally
the bodily changes associated with emotion in animals ; more
especially the effects produced by adrenalin.   He shewed that
the excitement produced by such emotions as fear or rage
affects the autonomic nervous system, and through the
impulses thus produced the adrenal glands are stimulated to
activity.   The adrenalin, which is secreted into the blood in
this way, stimulates the liver to produce sugar, increases
the force of muscular contraction, hastens the clotting of the
blood and increases blood pressure.   The body is thus placed
in a more favourable position and has a greater supply of
available energy to cope with some threatened danger. Exactly
similar results are produced by violent pain.   Now in a state
of nature fear or rage or pain would call for pugnacity, flight
and other violent exertion.   The body is thus automatically
regulated to cope with such situations.   Increased blood sugar,
an adapted circulation and rapid clotting are all favourable
to the preservation of the animal which can produce them.

At first sight this seems to support the theory of James
and Lange, that emotions are nothing but the reflex effect
in consciousness of such internal visceral changes.   But a
closer consideration shews this to be unfounded.   For, as far
as the visceral accompaniments are concerned, including in
these the secretions of the adrenal and other glands, there
appears to be no difference in bodily activity corresponding
to differences in the emotional state.   Both fear and rage,
for example, stop gastric digestion, and so will joy, if intense
enough.   As Professor Cannon says : " Any high degree of
excitement in the central nervous system, whether felt as
anger, terror, pain, anxiety, joy, grief or deep disgust is likely
to break over the threshold of the sympathetic system and
disturb the functions of all the organs which that system
innervates ".   Making due allowance for the physiological bias
of this statement, we may infer that there are no differences
in the reactions concerned or the effects produced which would
justify us in believing that emotions are the result of physiological action.   However various the emotions, the internal
bodily reactions are, as far as we can tell, exactly the same.

And moreover the visceral effects are almost entirely unconscious ; as we should expect them to be.

There are other unconscious effects associated with emotional states, but not confined to them any more than the visceral changes are. If two regions of the skin, one of which is rich in sweat glands, are connected through a galvanometer a deflection will ensue, indicating a difference of potential with a corresponding current. The current gradually subsides. But if any emotional excitement occurs, such as anger or annoyance, or any disagreeable or sudden sensation, such as a flash of light or a pin prick, the initial deflection increases, shewing that the potential difference has increased. The same result is produced if the person thinks of any past pleasant or unpleasant experience. A similar state of affairs is also brought about by any mental effort, such as working arithmetical problems, or producing word-associations. The phenomenon has received the name of the psycho-galvanic reflex. It has been explained by Dr D. Wechsler (7) as being due to the secretion of sweat. When the original current traverses the sweat glands there is an accumulation of ions at the membranes of the glands, producing an opposing electromotive force. Any emotional or mental effort which affects the body leads to renewed secretion, which sweeps away the polarized ions and so increases the difference of potential once again. The psycho-galvanic response thus indicates that the glandular mechanism is capable of adjustment to meet any demands which the body may make on it. It should be carefully noted that though the mechanism is entirely physiological it is nevertheless regulated by mental occurrences. So that even the metabolism of the tissues seems to be dependent on mental events ; thus providing a further illustration of what we learnt in earlier chapters of the primacy of mental forces in the mind-body relation.

As there is little physiological justification for assuming that emotions are determined by the products of endocrine glands, there is still less for supposing that temperaments are thus determined. We may, if we choose, suppose that temperament is somehow dependent on the bodily organism. What a psychological theory has to explain, however, is the varieties of temperament, and for this physiology offers no sort of help. For pathological cases give no manner of assistance in this difficulty, merely telling us what happens if the glands refuse to act. The position is exactly similar to what happens if a man is deprived of certain vitamins in his food. Sooner or later he will starve, but in the meantime he will become depressed or irritable and morose. Are we to say that a particular vitamin is the determiner of satisfaction or serenity because the lack of it in food results in the opposite emotions ?

Before endocrine glands were discovered the most generally held view was, as was previously said, that the nervous system was responsible for temperaments ; and this belief, as we have seen, may be combined with a belief in the efficacy of hormones for the same purpose. The first opinion, held by the physiologist Henle, was that the tone of the central nervous system determined temperament. But variations in tone, even if the conception was definite instead of being vague, would only account for variations within a single temperament ; if they accounted for anything at all in the mental sphere. And the explanation we require must account for varieties of temperament. It has been suggested that the intensity and speed of nervous impulses furnish the ground for differences of temperament and, in fact, Fouillée (8), in one of the best studies on the subject, uses this as a means of subdivision. We shall consider the validity of this idea later. Fouillée based his main classification, not on the nervous system or any particular set of organs but on the general cellular metabolism of the body. Metabolism has two phases, integration or anabolism and disintegration or katabolism. Where the former predominates we get the sensitive type, and predominance of the latter yields the active type of temperament. If these are combined with the nervous properties of intensity and speed of reaction, we get four main types of temperament, i.e. sensitives with quick reactions but feeble responses, sensitives with slow reactions but intense responses ; and so on for the active types. These are ingeniously related to the four classical varieties of temperament. Thus the sensitives with quick reactions are the sanguine type, the actives with prompt and intense reactions, the choleric type, and so forth. Fouillée is careful to point out, however, that the various types are not sharply separated ; " ce qui est introuvable c'est un pur sanguin, un pur nerveux, etc.". His final summary of the types shews the complete bankruptcy of all this physiological explanation. He says " Although we have taken the bilious as the relatively simple type of the ardent active, one can be active in another way, *i.e.* by the combination of the sanguine temperament with a temperament moderately nervous, and a well developed muscular system. The actives of the temperate regions, especially Celts and Gauls are in this category. Often also activity results from a mixture of sanguine, nervous and phlegmatic temperaments ; this resultant being common amongst English, Dutch and Germans." The literature of temperaments is overloaded with suggestions of this kind about national psychology combined with descriptions of various kinds of character ; each writer finding a confirmation of his views in such character studies. If activity can be produced by any combination of temperaments we like to choose, of what value is the classification ?

The division of personalities into two main types, the sensitives and the actives, was first suggested by Ribot. (9) He based himself purely on psychological considerations, regarding mental life as an alternation of receptive and reactive states. Those in whom the receptive states were prominent were the sensitives. In them sensibility predominated, and they were emotional, being peculiarly susceptible to pleasurable or painful impressions, meditative or contemplative and timid. In strong contrast to these were the actives, in whom the will predominated. These were rich in energy, bold and ready to face obstacles. In opposition to the former, who were inclined to pessimism, these were born optimists. Ribot worked out this distinction of types in great detail, regarding it as the first *fundamentum divisionis* of character.

William James (10) popularized this division into types, and in his usual vivid and picturesque style called them the ' tender-minded ' and the ' tough-minded ' respectively. The tender-minded are distinguished by a predominating interest in their own experiences or the inner life, whilst the tough-minded lay most stress on the outer world or objective reality. He found this contrast of temperaments, as he described it, in philosophers, as rationalists and empiricists ; in literature, as the classics and the romantics, and in most other spheres of activity. James was quite aware that such a sharp division of types was " to a certain extent arbitrary ", as every sort of permutation and combination was found in real people, yet he was carried away by his own eloquence. As soon as we take this distinction, which is ultimately founded on the difference between the emotions and the will, too seriously, we begin to find ourselves involved in contradictions. As a popular mode of classification it is admirable, but as representing real temperamental types, which is what James imagined it to be, it will not bear investigation. Ribot, as we saw above, described the sensitives (the tender-minded) as born pessimists, whereas for James they were exactly the opposite, being the true-blue optimists. This is the kind of irreconcilable opposition which has pervaded the doctrine of temperaments from its inception, and justifies Mr Shand's remark that it has never been lifted out of that loose and popular status to which its original defects condemned it.

Nevertheless the tendency to a bifurcation of temperamental types seems to have an irresistible attraction for psychologists and has been ably supported by Dr C. G. Jung. (11) He approves of James' classification, and finding a similar twofold division in other writers he concludes that it represents a real temperamental distinction. His own conviction was founded, in the first instance, on a study of morbid psychology, being thus in the true line of descent from the ancient doctrine. Through the ages, from the time of Hippocrates and Galen to the present day, the doctrine of temperaments has rested on three pillars, bodily organization, pathological data, and a belief in opposites. Dr Jung finds his opposites in the distinction between sufferers from hysteria and dementia praecox respectively. At the outset of the disease, the hysterical patient exhibits exaggerated emotivity, thus recalling

Ribot's sensitives, whilst the dement shews extreme apathy towards his environment. The energy of the one has a centrifugal tendency ; whilst in dementia praecox its tendency is centripetal.

A remarkable change occurs, however, when the illness is fully established ; for it is the nature of mental disease to be ' contrary ' and to try to compensate for what it most lacks. Jung has vividly described what is supposed to occur. " In the hysteric the libido [energy] is always hampered in its movements of expansion and forced to regress upon itself ; one observes that such individuals cease to partake in the common life, are wrapped up in their phantasies, keep their beds, or are unable to live outside their sick rooms, etc. The precocious dement, on the contrary, during the incubation of his illness turns away from the outer world in order to withdraw into himself ; but when the period of morbid compensation arrives, he seems constrained to draw attention to himself, and to force himself upon the notice of those around him, by his extravagant, insupportable, or directly aggressive conduct."

He uses the terms ' extraversion ' and ' introversion ' to describe the direction that the vital energy takes in the two cases. A person is an extravert when his fundamental attraction is to the outer or objective world, which alone he regards as having value. The introvert, on the other hand, ignores the outer world and exalts his own inner life, so that his intense concentration on his own feelings makes them the centre of his universe. This opposition of introversion and extraversion, which characterizes dementia praecox and hysteria respectively, is believed to be but an exaggerated form of two normal temperaments, in accordance with the view that mental disease simply brings into prominence what is previously latent in the normal mind. Inasmuch as the distinction of types between introverts and extraverts rests on psychological grounds alone and is entirely divorced from physiological considerations, it has the same merit as Ribot's classification of the temperaments of men. Valuable and suggestive as the classification undoubtedly is, however, as soon as an attempt is made to apply it in detail it leads to the usual contradictions. Thus Jung says " the introvert uses his thought as the function of adaptation, thinking beforehand how he shall act ; whilst the extravert, on the contrary, feels his way into the object by acting. In extreme cases the one limits himself to thinking and observing, and the other to feeling and acting. It is true that the introvert feels also, very deeply ; indeed, almost too deeply ; that is why an English investigator has gone so far as to describe his as ' the emotional type.' True, the emotion is there, but it all remains inside, and the more passionate and deeper his feeling is, the quieter is his outward demeanour. As the proverb puts it, ' Still waters run deep.' Similarly, the extravert *thinks* also, but that likewise mostly inside, whilst his feelings visibly go outside, that is why he is held to be full of feeling, while the introvert is considered cold and dry." Any attempt to reconcile these types with those of James, to which they are supposed to correspond, is hopeless, for each has some of the characteristics which are supposed to be the peculiar property of the other.

The most suggestive study of the temperaments we owe to Dr E. Kretschmer (12) and is to be found in his work on *Physique and Character*, the title of which shews that the conception of temperament is still sought in the bodily organism. On the basis of physical measurements, combined with close observation of the shape of the features, the disposition of the hair on the body, the texture of the skin, the functioning of the glands and so forth, he distinguishes three main types of physique. The poorest in bodily qualities are asthenics, who are lean but of average height, with ill-developed muscles, narrow shoulders, flat chest, poor skin and blood. The finest are the athletic, with strong development of skeleton, musculature and skin, and above the average height and strength. The third type are the pyknic, medium in height or short, with rounded figures and protuberant stomachs, soft limbs and massive neck. Now Kraepelin distinguished two sharply differentiated types of insanity, the manic-depressive or circular type and schizophrenia or dementia praecox. By studying the physique of asylum patients suffering from these insanities, Kretschmer concluded that there was biological affinity between circular insanity and the pyknic type on the one hand, and between schizophrenia and asthenics and athletics on the other.

The modern conception of mental disease, as we previously stated, regards it not as something suddenly arising, but as inherent in the constitutional make-up of the patient. A person destined to suffer from one of the above types of insanity has a mental constitution in which the seeds of his disease may be discovered by a close observer. The early histories of the circular type shew, according to Kretschmer, people who are sociable, genial, humorous, soft-hearted, but with a tendency towards easy depression. Whereas the psychopathic constitution of the future schizophrene is marked, especially at puberty, by traits of unsociableness, reserve, eccentricity, lack of humour, indifference and dullness. It will be observed that there is an approximation here to the extraverts and introverts of Jung.

So far, so good ; but all this refers to abnormal people who by their very nature would be bound to display outstanding characteristics, since otherwise they would not be abnormal. Nevertheless it is maintained that the same characteristics are to be observed in normal folk, and that there are two strongly marked normal temperaments, cyclothymes and schizothymes, who can be distinguished by their general physique, and fall respectively into the pyknic or the athletic and asthenic classes. Cyclothymes, like their unfortunate analogues amongst the insane, oscillate between exalted and depressed moods. Their psychic tempo is wavy or smooth ; and this is characteristic, too, of their responses to stimuli which are smooth, adequate and natural. As a contrast to these, schizothymes are, as regards their emotional life, either extremely sensitive or blunt. They have a jerky temperamental curve and their reactions to stimuli are inadequate, being either restrained or inhibited. These then are the two diverse temperaments exhibited by normal people ; and it is easy to see that the variety of traits may yield almost any combination of emotional life we like to make. That is to say, it is possible by arranging and rearranging the above qualities to draw any psychic portrait we please.

It is suggested that these two types of temperament depend ultimately on two hormone groups, of which the one determines one kind of physique and the other group the other. This has been very clearly stated by Kretschmer, who says : " It is not a great step to the suggestion that the chief normal types of temperament, cyclothymes and schizothymes, are determined with regard to their physical correlates [*i.e.* bodily physique] by similar parallel activity on the part of the secretions, by which we naturally do not mean merely the internal secretions in the narrow sense, but the whole chemistry of the blood, in as much as it is also conditioned to a very important degree, *e.g.* by the great intestinal glands, and ultimately by every tissue of the body. We can imagine provisionally that a man's temperament is dependent on two great chemical hormone groups, of which the one corresponds to the cyclothymic type, and the other to the schizothymic. . . . In the present incomplete state of our knowledge, we must not lay any great weight on these theoretical suggestions."

In so far as this physiological view refers temperament to the complete bodily organism instead of to one particular set of organs, it is an undoubted advance on earlier ideas. Nevertheless, being founded on a physiological basis, it is subject to the criticisms already made : and, moreover, the statistical evidence on which it rests is not very thorough. Further, when the attempt is made to apply the concept to actual people, the reservations, rearrangements, combinations and contradictions which ensue suggest, as was stated above, that the types are artifacts. This is admitted by Kretschmer, who states that " Temperament has for us no well-defined meaning, but it is a heuristic notion, the breadth of whose field of reference we have not yet determined." It would save a good deal of controversy if all writers on temperament were equally cautious.

In fact, as Mr A. F. Shand (13) has ingeniously remarked, what is the use of all such explanations if we do not know what we have to explain ? Let us, then, attempt to clear our ideas, if we can, as to what we mean by temperament. This can only be done by first considering what is meant by individuality or character. "What is fundamental in character" said Ribot, "is instincts, tendencies, impulses, desires, sentiments ; all that and nothing but that." Character thus expresses what is most subjective, most intimate in a human being, and its hidden source is to be found in the emotions and the will. But the various constituents by themselves, however blended, do not form character. What is essential in order to constitute character, is unity and stability, or acting in a manner consistent with oneself. The various desires, sentiments, or what not, must all be convergent, or, at all events, consistent with one another. A mere collection of instincts, desires, impulses, etc., is merely a collection. Unless they form a well-knit unity acting in a single direction, there is nothing worthy of the name of character. The unity also must persist, that is to say, there is no character without a certain measure of stability, or the persistence of unity over a period of time. It is quite true, of course, that characters all of a piece and stable over a prolonged period are rare, or rather ideal ; yet there is no doubt that this is the idea we have in mind when we use the concept of character ; and it is by a criterion of this kind that our judgments on character and personality are formed. A considerable number of people have neither the unity nor the stability demanded by the concept, *i.e.* they are amorphous or unstable. Such character as they possess is plastic and they are the sport of circumstances. Their social environment does their willing and acting for them, as it were ; they are not voices but echoes. Their careers are determined by chance or are determined for them, for of themselves they are quite indeterminate. Now it is within this general concept of character that temperament is usually distinguished.

Between the action of the physical and social environment on us and our reactions thereto, there is an intermediary, a sort of affective-conative refractive medium. Just as a ray of white light traversing different media will produce different colours, so the same set of impressions will give rise to different responses in different individuals. In so far as such responses are supposed to be innate and dependent on the physical constitution, so far is our temperament said to be involved. It determines the tone, the nature, the tempo and direction of our emotional responses. Temperament is thus a part of character, that fund of tendencies to respond which expresses innate constitution as opposed to the mass of tendencies to action which are acquired by experience from the physical or social environment. As Fouillée has pithily expressed it : " nos impulsions aveugles et nos goûts instinctifs tiennent à notre temperament ; nos amours, à notre caractère."

Temperament thus refers, in the main, to what is inherited as opposed to what is acquired. It would, no doubt, be difficult to draw a sharp line between the two, but this objection may be ignored, for the present, whilst we consider what evidence there is for the belief that temperament is innate. It was Francis Galton (14) who first suggested that mental and moral qualities might be inherited, just as bodily qualities were. He obtained careful accounts of twins, getting their parents or other near relatives to fill up a questionnaire regarding their resemblances and differences. He concluded that such differences as were found, constituted a difference in key-note, and not in melody. Out of eighty pairs of twins he found only two cases of strong physical resemblances accompanied by mental or moral diversity. In many cases the twins were reared exactly alike till adolescence, and then the conditions of their lives changed : nevertheless, the mental resemblances continued unaltered in the majority, and their temperamental qualities were also apparently the same. There is also some slight evidence to shew that identical twins suffer from the same periodical depressions or melancholia, even when they live far apart and undergo very dissimilar experiences.

C. B. Davenport (15) studied the question whether violent temper was inherited, by getting histories of wayward girls in institutions. From an examination of the family records of these girls he concluded that the tendency to outbursts of temper, whether associated with epilepsy or hysteria or

K

not, was a positive dominant trait in the Mendelian sense ; and tends to appear in a considerable proportion of children of an affected person. Davenport calculated the different combinations that would result on Mendelian lines from the presence or absence of a hyperkinetic and a hypokinetic factor. He then investigated family records of ninety unselected families in institutions and found that the calculated numbers agreed with the records. From this he inferred that there is a factor in the inheritance of a person which induces an excited condition and another which yields depression, and that temperament is " determined " by this pair of hereditary factors. The evidence is not very convincing. It is far too subjective and capable of varying interpretations, and many of the families were undoubtedly abnormal, as all were institutional cases. In addition no distinction was made between mood, temper and temperament, thus confusing the issue.

To understand temperament we must distinguish it from temper ; for, as was said above, what is the use of discussing whether temperament is dependent on the bodily organism if we don't know what we mean by temperament. Now the fact of the matter is that we don't know scientifically what we mean by temperament, and that the classical view, together with its modern revisions, is based on erroneous assumptions. By temperament is ordinarily meant, as was previously said, that part of a man's native constitution which has reference to his affective and volitional life, and is somehow dependent on his bodily organism. The latter part of this belief we have already considered and it remains to discover the grounds for the former portion. Different people experience specific emotions, such as anger, in very different ways. They are, as it were, attuned to different keys with regard to these emotions. Thus an angry man may, with reference to his anger, be violent, sullen, peevish and so forth ; and similarly with regard to any other definite emotion. In popular discourse such variations are described as differences of temper ; this term having a peculiar connection with the emotion of anger. Now the tempers of men are subject to great variations in the course of their lives, and the evidence for the inheritance of tempers, which we referred to above, is but meagre. The relation of temper to some particular emotion is parallel to the relation of temperament to emotional life in general. Temperament is usually considered a more comprehensive term, referring to the totality of a man's emotions and conative experiences, being the keynote of all such experiences. Just as with regard to the emotion of fear, for example, a person may have a timorous or rash temper, so with respect to his whole emotional life, it is asserted that he may be sanguine or phlegmatic or cyclothymic or possessed of some other temperament.

As Mr A. F. Shand has pointed out, in a most acute study of temperaments in his book on the *Foundations of Character*, the very definite assumption involved in the doctrine of temperaments has no foundation in fact. If we take any pair of contrasted temperaments, such as the sanguine and the bilious, all authorities are agreed that the distinguishing mark of the former type is superficiality of the feelings and its consequences. Their emotions have neither stability nor depth ; in contrast to the bilious, who display depth and stability, which enables them to pursue a single purpose with unswerving fidelity. What these metaphorical expressions mean is that the emotions of the sanguine are evanescent, whilst those of the bilious are lasting. But there is no reason whatever to suppose that this is true of all their emotions ; and the vast majority of people are surely ' contradictory ', being stable in some of their feelings and unstable in others. With respect to such people, therefore, the conception of temperament is inapplicable. A man may have an irascible temper, being easily roused to anger which soon passes off, but he need not be correspondingly hasty and superficial in his other feelings. As these facts are too obvious to be ignored, those who adhere to the doctrine of temperaments have been forced, as we have seen, to recognize ' mixed types ' ; which they mix according to fancy. The pure types are simply literary exaggerations of one aspect of the temperaments of all normal people. Human nature is too variable to be restricted to ' types ', except for crude popular purposes of classification, and no matter how numerous the permutations and combinations, the great bulk of human beings are too fluid to have any fixed boundaries.

We have seen that temperament is a wider concept than temper, since the traits which constitute a man's temperament are supposed to colour his whole emotional and volitional life. For example, intensity or speed of reaction is ascribed to the man of nervous temperament and is contrasted with the slowness or apathy of the phlegmatic man. But we have been led to suspect the validity of such sweeping assertions as that a certain trait pervades the whole of a person's reactions. In matters of this kind general observation is hardly sufficient and it is desirable, on scientific grounds, to get experimental data. Unfortunately the testing of temperamental traits is in its extreme infancy, but such investigations as have been made lead to the conclusion that the belief in general traits is unwarranted. Quickness and slowness can be readily measured by a variety of tests, and when this is done it turns out that the majority of persons are found to be inconsistent in different tests. But other qualities can hardly be measured, especially as we do not know what we are looking for.

Nevertheless an attempt has been made to get statistical information about such qualities by the employment of the Downey will-temperament tests. These attempt to tackle the difficulty by testing a person's power to modify certain habitual activities such as those employed in handwriting. By interfering with a man's stable habits it is hoped to bring to light his temperamental characteristics. There are a dozen of such tests arranged in three groups which are supposed to discover speed of reaction, forcefulness and decisiveness, and carefulness and persistence of response respectively. Such tests have been applied to numbers of students with the result that the intercorrelations between the tests of any one group are found, for reasons which are now clear to us, to be very low or negative. Mr D. W. Oates (16) made a careful statistical investigation of the tests as applied to boys in his school, whose character traits were well known, and concluded that there was no indication of general factors of speed, aggressiveness, persistence, etc. He states, and it is a conclusion that might have been anticipated, that certain so-called temperamental traits may affect a person's dealing with a limited group of situations but will not be evident outside these. " When we say a boy is energetic, keen, careful and trustworthy, we describe his tendencies with a certain degree of accuracy. But this is only approximately an accurate description, for he is probably not always energetic and careful, nor is he equally keen and trustworthy in the face of different situations." This is a headmaster's view, and though all these are not traits of the same category, the opinion is certainly valid as regards temperamental traits.

It is, therefore, evident that the attempt to account for temperament on the grounds of internal secretions, or in more general physiological terms, is impossible. For the hormones, whatever their function, can hardly be selective in dealing with different situations. Since there is no general factor at the back of all temperamental traits, but at most group factors, it would be passing strange if a man's physical constitution should determine that he is to be violent and aggressive in his politics but calm and subdued in his family relations.

If we attempt to summarize all the evidence, we are inevitably led to the very modest conclusion that everybody is possessed of a mixed temperament. Perhaps even this modest result is somewhat hasty and must be hedged about with reservations. The various qualities which are said to distinguish differences of temperament are not characteristics of well-marked types of people, but qualities of character which are possessed by all persons in varying degrees at different times, and shewn in different circumstances. But this conclusion, too, is probably overhasty, and we ought to say that the varous temperaments are a set of adjectives by which we try to describe certain aspects of character which are emotional or volitional as opposed to intellectual.

The attempts to justify the physiological view of temperament have brought all the outstanding physiological discoveries into the field, with one exception. I am very much surprised that nobody has yet attempted to base the varieties of temperament on differences of chronaxy in the nerves. In studying the nervous system we saw that the attempt to isolate one organ or set of organs and to consider their functions apart from the rest of the organism is no longer tenable. A collection of organs is not an organism, any more than a collection of faculties is a mind. If we admit this, we see the error of trying to find specific mental characters in particular bodily happenings, whether nervous or glandular or what not. Accordingly Kretschmer is justified in directing his attention to the whole of man's bodily constitution, his physique, his glandular secretions, his blood, his nervous system and the rest. But, if this is done, then the relation of temperament to bodily constitution is but another name for the general relation of body to mind. Our examination has shewn that the assumption that the relation is one in which the mind somehow mirrors the bodily constitution is not justified by the evidence. We are inevitably led to the conclusion that temperament is a conception valuable to the novelist and dramatist in their delineations of character, but unsuitable for scientific treatment.

Laboratory workers and practical investigators have been driven to the same conclusion, as perhaps might have been anticipated. Thus Mr P. E. Vernon (17) who worked with the Downey tests abandoned them in favour of observing the behaviour of his subjects when they played a variety of parlour games, on the ground that the personality or temperament of an individual is something qualitative and subjective which cannot be interpreted in objective terms nor measured. To describe or understand a man's temperament we need the outlook and method of approach not of the scientist but of the dramatist. Intuitive emotional insight into character is the best equipment for understanding temperamental or personality traits and neither physiological data nor any other scientific equipment can be a substitute for this. The point of view of the artist is the only one that is appropriate to dealing with character qualities. " Ein guter Psycholog muss nicht nur ein Gelehrter, sondern auch ein Künstler sein."

In order to illustrate the impassable gulf separating the scientific and artistic treatment of the matter I will end this chapter with a description of personality, from which the temperaments are but abstractions. The description is from a character study by Miss R. Langbridge. (18) " The word ' personality ' is as difficult to define as ' charm '. It is not the same as individuality, which is a blend of hereditary characteristics with those begotten on heredity by environment. Personality may be called the quintessence of individuality, as scent may be described as the personality of every individual flower. And just as no two flowers give forth exactly the same scent, and as certain scents attract certain insects and people, and repel others, so personality is differentiated in every human being, attractive, or repulsive to other human beings, and, like the scent of flowers, is more distinctive in the open air of freedom than when it is cabined and confined.

" Personality is largely born of freedom : freedom for full expression of the individual likes and dislikes, whims, fancies and indulgencies, for it is an olla podrida of all these fleeting and elusive matters, and, in analysis, a frail elusive thing, like scent itself."

If anybody will contrast this sketch with the analytical descriptive accounts given by scientists or with the physiological investigations to which we have referred, he will immediately realize that he is faced with two totally different universes of ideas. In the one he is in touch with reality, whereas the other is concerned with dubious abstractions. We may safely conclude that temperament, like personality, can only be adequately understood from the artistic standpoint.

CHAPTER VII

MENTAL ENERGY

OUR account of the doctrine of temperaments has revealed the fact that the various types into which neurologists have divided human beings have, in several cases, been distinguished by variations in the energy of the nervous system. It behoves us, therefore, to examine the doctrine of energy from the psychological aspect. The first attempt to introduce the concept of mental energy into psychology was made by Francis Galton in his *Inquiries into human Faculty*. He defined energy as the capacity for labour and regarded it as an indication of superior mental ability. The higher races were more endowed with it than the lower, and leaders of intellectual thought had more energy than ordinary men, having inherited it from their ancestors. On the other hand, those of a lower mentality had less energy, which explained why idiots were feeble and listless. In any scheme of eugenics he thought that energy was the most important quality to favour as it was eminently transmissible to descendants. However, he does not seem to have regarded energy as much more than a synonym for general vitality and vigour ; in the sense in which we speak of a healthy man as being energetic.

Modern psychology goes much further than this and makes such abundant use of the doctrine of mental energy that it is desirable to examine the concept closely in order to see what it involves. A concept which purports to convert psychology from an outworn static science to a dynamic study ought to have the merit of being at once precise, definite and intelligible. It should be supported by experiment or, at least, by accurate observation ; or if it is derived from the physical sciences it must conform to the modern physical views of energy. In all these respects the doctrine of mental energy seems conspicuously to have failed to live up to its scientific reputation. The thesis I wish to maintain is that the concept of mental energy as used by modern psychologists is based on analogies which have ceased to have any explanatory value. " The progress of science," says Professor Whitehead (1) " has now reached a turning point. The stable foundations of physics have broken up. . . . The old foundations of scientific thought are becoming unintelligible. Time, space, matter, material, ether, electricity, mechanism, organism, configuration, structure, pattern, function, all require reinterpretation. What is the sense of talking about a mechanical explanation when you do not know what you mean by mechanics ? "

In the above enumeration of physical concepts it is startling to find the omission of any reference to energy. The explanation of this gap seems to be given in the subsequent statement (2) that " the physicist's energy is obviously an abstraction." But such an abstraction will not serve the purpose of psychological explanation which demands for a dynamic psychology something concrete, possessing motive power, which no abstraction can provide. An abstract energy, devoid of motive force and lacking concrete reality is an admirable mathematical idea, but to change the above query : What is the use of talking about dynamical psychology in terms of energy when the energy has no power to do anything ?

If we leave physical ideas on one side, for the present, the obvious place to seek support for the concept of mental energy is in the phenomena of fatigue. For, at first sight, the relation between energy and fatigue seems as direct as that between capital and expenditure. If the notion of mental energy cannot explain mental fatigue it is difficult to see how it can justify itself elsewhere.

Investigations on fatigue have usually been devoted to the estimation of the diminution of capacity to carry out a given task before and after a period of activity. Thus a person first performs a set task and then works steadily for a measured period of time. At the end of this period he is again given a task exactly similar to the first ; and his lowered capacity in its performance is taken as a measure of his fatiguability.

A slight variant of this procedure consists in estimating the subject's capacity in the morning, and again in the evening after his ordinary day's work. In the laboratory, the method used is somewhat different. The subject undertakes a piece of work, such as multiplying numbers, or adding figures, or crossing out letters ; and the amount of his performance is gauged at equal intervals. The effects of fatigue are then sought in the amount of his performance during each of these intervals. As, however, practice increases the capacity of the subject and consequently the amount he is able to perform in a given time interval, various devices have been used to counterbalance this effect. The favourite procedure is to give the subject so much preliminary practice in the task that he reaches the limit of his capacity. After this point of saturation has been reached, any diminution in capacity is attributed to the effects of fatigue.

Another device is to measure the number of errors in a set task, or in a given time, after eliminating as before, the increase of accuracy which comes about as the result of practice. For industrial purposes the number of accidents or the amount of spoiled work has been employed as a measure of fatigue ; but since an accident or spoiled work is due to some error, this method does not differ fundamentally from the one just considered. All of the above methods have been employed to indicate and measure both bodily and mental fatigue ; but ideas on mental fatigue are very hazy and the two are usually mixed up in the same investigation.

Instead of making a frontal attack on the problem a few investigators have tried to carry the position by a side manœuvre. This has arisen, in the main, from the unsatisfactory and conflicting evidence obtained by the aforementioned methods ; since the results have been in many cases mutually contradictory. For this reason measures of sensory processes, such as visual or auditory acuity, or sensitivity to pain, or some other physiological function, such as blood pressure, have been employed as measures to indicate fatigue. The sensory acuity of a person is tested before and after a day's labour and the decrease of acuity is taken as an indication of fatigue. The assumption underlying such a procedure seems to be that as energy is employed in the labour there will be less available for other purposes, such as visual or auditory activity. I have called this a side attack as the measure of fatigue is sought in a function far removed from that employed in doing the day's work. No doubt the investigators have assumed, more or less unconsciously, that each person has a definite fund or reservoir of energy. If he uses it up in doing physical or mental work there will be less available for seeing or hearing, or any other sensory function whatever.

Professor Wm. McDougall and Professor C. Spearman have dragged this unconscious assumption into the light of day and make considerable use of the hypothesis of a reserve supply or fund of energy. The former employs it to elucidate and support his theory of instincts and the latter regards it as a cardinal point in his doctrine of the two factors in Intelligence. Nevertheless, no attempt is made to define the notion of psycho-physical or mental energy, and it is hard to find out what is the evidence which leads to the assumption of a reservoir in which it is kept ; for both undoubtedly believe that it is somehow ' stored ' in the nervous system.

The clearest statement on the matter is that of Professor McDougall (3), who says : " The essence of instinctive activity seems to be such liberation and direction of energy, which we may best speak of as psycho-physical energy. We are naturally inclined to suppose that it is a case of conversion of potential energy stored in the tissues in chemical form, into the free and active form, kinetic or electric or what not ; and probably this view is correct ". He then goes on to consider whether each instinct has its own store of energy or whether they all draw upon " a common store of reserve energy." And he gives his adherence to the latter view : " Each instinct," he says, " is in part a sluice-gate in the system of barriers which dams back the energy liberated in the afferent side of the nervous system ; on the stimulation of the instinct . . . the sluice-gate swings open and makes the efferent channels of the instinct the principal outlet." He tells us that the sluice-gates are situated in the *optic thalamus*, but does not state where the reservoir is located.

Professor C. Spearman does not leave us in the dark with regard to the locality. He informs us (4) that his 'general factor' is "something of the nature of an 'energy' or 'power' which serves in common the whole cortex (or possibly, even the whole nervous system)." He does not employ sluice-gates but 'engines' to drain the reservoir; each engine corresponding to a 'specific factor', being the group of neurones specially serving the particular kind of operation. "These neural groups would thus function as alternate 'engines' into which the common supply of 'energy' could be alternatively distributed." In any given individual the quantity of energy is stated to be constant, for, "the said constancy manifests itself in the fact that the occurrence of any one process tends to diminish the others, whilst conversely the fact of any one process ceasing tends to augment the others." (4)

The brain as we have learnt from physiology is a very complicated, discriminative and responsive organ ; but it has one function which is more remarkable than any which the neurologists have been able to discover, or, even, most of them to conceive. Professor Spearman describes it thus : "The brain may be regarded (pending further information) as able to switch the bulk of its energy from any one to any other group of neurons." (4) But what the cortex does is not to switch on energy accumulated in certain hypothetical 'centres' but to co-ordinate nervous impulses or to shunt them in certain directions. The idea that certain groups of neurons have a fund of energy at their disposal on which they are able to cash drafts is not borne out by a study of cerebral physiology. "The doctrine of nervous energy," says K. S. Lashley, "as derived by analogy with forms of physical energy, seems precluded by what we know of the nature of nerve conduction. If, as seems probable from studies of the refractory period of nerve, the response of the neuron is momentary and is followed by a quick return to the resting state after every excitation, there can be no general fund of nervous energy capable of accumulation and diversion into various activities." (5) The modern view of the function of the brain has been clearly stated by Dr H. Head. (6) " Whenever a primitive function is rendered more perfect and is given a wider range of purposive adaptation, the structures which are primarily responsible for its existence become linked up with those on a higher anatomical plane of the nervous system. But many of the more mechanical processes and the actual force expended may still be furnished by the lower functional levels. No fresh ' energy ' is generated by this higher integration, but the response gains in freedom ; it can be more closely regulated according to the needs of the moment and brought into harmony with the reaction of the organism as a whole. This is the purpose of that series of complex integrative changes ". It is a mistake to suppose that there is any point-to-point correspondence between the production of a psychical act, such as solving a problem, and the activity of any particular group of neurons. For this is simply the old faculty psychology translated into neurological terms. There is, therefore, no physiological warrant for believing in the theory of a fund of energy switched from place to place in the cortex. What the brain does to nervous impulses is to act like a complicated series of railway points. If I lift up my arm to ward off a threatening blow, all the energy employed in this process comes from oxidation of material in the muscle fibres themselves and none of it from the central nervous system. The brain ensures that the impression on my retina shall bring into activity my arm rather than my leg, but it does not supply the energy needed for the activity. So, when I am hungry and smell food saliva begins to flow, but the energy for this activity comes entirely from the salivary glands and the same result would be produced by stimulating the facial nerve even if it were severed from the brain. All that the cortex does is to set the points leading the impulse from the olfactory nerves to the glands, but it supplies no energy for the secretion.

Psychologists have long contracted the bad habit of inventing a physiology to suit their purpose. But they are not very much to blame in this, since much of what passes for physiology amongst neurologists is pure psychology clothed with a garment of neurons to hide its physiological nakedness. Thus, for example, the law of association of ideas was begotten originally by introspection ; and, indeed, it is difficult to see what other method was or is possible. Yet Hartley, in the middle of the eighteenth century, finding it in its bare psychological state, invested it with physiological clothing which it could very well have dispensed with. Ever since then people have assumed that physiologists discovered the law by finding chains of neurones in the cerebral cortex functioning together, or different centres rousing one another to action. Thomas Brown, at the beginning of the nineteenth century tried to tear off the covering and display the real psychological law, naked and unadorned. (7) But, to the great detriment of psychology, the attempt was unsuccessful.

Modern neurologists simply repeat these theories but much more cautiously in some cases. Thus Professor C. J. Herrick (8) says " That which we *know subjectively* as the association of ideas *may*, in a somewhat similar way, be *pictured* as involving neurologically the discharge of nervous energy in the cortex between two systems of neurons which have in some previous experience been physiologically united in some cortical reaction " (italics mine). He adds, however, that " it should be emphasized that the mechanism of association here suggested is purely theoretical; we have little [? no] scientific evidence regarding the details of such physiological processes ". This laudable caution is due to the fact that he, unlike some neurologists, is quite familiar with psychological theory and he is amply justified in saying that " it is possible to develop a really scientific introspective psychology in which abstraction is made from all of these (physiological) mechanisms and the individual experiences alone are studied as given in consciousness ". It is worthy of note that Hartley based his physiological psychology on the *function* of the nerves, not on their anatomy. His disciples, the present-day physiological psychologists, with less insight, have tried to find the law of association in the nervous *structure*, *i.e.* in chains or systems of neurons. Hartley adopted the Newtonian dynamics and wrote entirely of vibrations, thus using the most modern physics of his day.

For him neural vibrations were the essential underlying facts both of sensation and ideation. If we must adopt physical analogies in psychology it is as well to follow Hartley's lead and to use the latest available ideas.

The psychologist who has made the most consistent attempt to do this is undoubtedly Dr C. G. Jung who has devoted a long essay to the subject of " Psychical Energy " in which he tries to shew that there is a complete analogy between this conception and that of physical energy. (9) He definitely repudiates the notion that psychical energy can be transformed into physical energy or *vice vérsa* ; and maintains that the energic standpoint in psychology demands that the psyche should be regarded as a closed system. Unless this can be done, he says, the analogy completely breaks down. Moreover he sees clearly, what his followers always ignore, that " the applicability of the energic standpoint to psychology rests *exclusively* upon the question whether a *quantitative* evaluation of psychic energy is possible " (my italics). He asserts emphatically that this is possible " because our minds possess what is in fact an exceedingly well developed evaluating system, namely, the *system of psychological values*. Values are indices of amounts of energy " (his italics).

Such a method of securing a quantitative estimate is, at first sight, somewhat startling but there is nothing inherently absurd in the attempt. It can only be judged by its success. After all we can, within limits, estimate colour intensities by the eye and auditory intensities by the ear. And Jung thinks that we can weigh, in the same way, our psychological contents one against the other and thus determine their comparative intensities. He agrees that the relative value-intensities of such different contents as, for instance, " the comparison of the value of a scientific concept and a feeling impression " is a difficult process ; but thinks it is a possible one. Anybody who can follow him and make this comparison is justified in employing the energic standpoint. I find it utterly impossible even to understand what the comparison means.

Now it is manifest that such subjective comparison could

only be conceived as possible for conscious processes, but as Jung is a protagonist of unconscious processes he is compelled to search for some other measure for these latter. Such an objective measure, he contends, is to be found in the 'complexes.' A complex is supposed to be an emotionally-toned system consisting of a nuclear or feeling element and a number of constellated associations. The nucleus is regarded as the bearer of the energy by which it is enabled to attract to itself the cloud of associations. Or in Jung's words " the constellating power of the nuclear element corresponds to its value intensity, which in turn represents its energy ". This energy can be estimated by the number of constellations which a nucleus can command, by the frequency and intensity of the ' complex-indicators ' such as lapses of speech or failures of memory, and finally by the strength of the feeling reactions such as those studied by the psycho-galvanic reflex. All these are obviously indirect means of evaluating the energy of the unconscious. But Jung believes that we have, in addition, a direct instinct by which we become aware of the least variation of an emotional character in others. So that what it comes to is this : we can measure our own conscious energy and our neighbour's unconscious energy, both by a direct method.

It will be seen that, leaving on one side the ambiguities in the term ' value ', the cogency of all this is dependent on the logical validity of the argument from analogy. According to J. S. Mill (10) the value of an analogical argument which infers one resemblance from other resemblances, without any antecedent evidence of a connection between them, depends upon certain very definite conditions. There must be a large number of ascertained resemblances, compared first with the amount of ascertained differences, and next with the extent of the unexplored region of unascertained properties. It follows that where the resemblance is very great, the ascertained difference very small and our knowledge of the subject matter tolerably extensive the argument from analogy is a good one.

It is the great merit of Dr Jung that he makes a really serious attempt to find such resemblances and to shew that our knowledge of the psyche is sufficiently wide to warrant the analogy between psychical and physical energy. Psychical energy or libido is a part of life energy and is not exclusively sexual, as Freud supposed, but is the general urge to activity of any sort. As there is actual and potential energy in the physical world so in the psyche actual energy appears as instinct, wishing, affect, attention, etc., whilst potential energy is to be sought in acquisitions, dispositions, aptitudes, attitudes, etc. But the resemblances must also extend to the attested quantitative aspects, such as the conservation of energy and entropy. Dr Jung does not shrink from the comparison but welcomes it. He says, rightly, that the use of the concept of psychical energy without these quantitative resemblances would be valueless. Accordingly he maintains that the disappearance of a quantum of libido must be followed by the appearance of a corresponding quantity in another form. Whenever a conscious value disappears we must look for a surrogate elsewhere. This is not so difficult as we might suppose, for the psycho-analyst always has the unconscious to fall back upon in all his explanations. " If the analyst is successful in tracing back symptoms to the hidden content of the unconscious, it can usually be shewn that the libido-sum which was lost from the conscious has developed a structure in the unconscious which, despite all differences, has not a few features in common with those conscious contents that were deprived of their energy."

Let us suppose a case which psycho-analysts assert occurs constantly, namely that an emotional event happening in childhood produces far-reaching effects extending over the greater part of life. A good example is the case of claustrophobia reported by Dr Rivers, in which a terrifying experience at the age of four produced stammering and horror of closed places lasting for more than a quarter of a century. What we are asked to believe is that the potential energy accumulated during the minute or two of the obnoxious experience was the exact quantitative equivalent of all the actual symptoms and emotions and horrible dreams which the patient suffered over this prolonged period. The libido released during all this time was laid up in a single buried complex of high explosive potentiality. Is this possible or even conceivable ?

So much for the conservation of energy. There remains the question of entropy. According to this doctrine a closed energic system gradually tends to equalize its differences of intensity so that further change is precluded. If the analogy is to hold, a similar phenomenon must be observable in the psyche, for it too is, as we saw, a closed system. This is supposed to happen whenever we attain a fixed and unchanging attitude after violent mental conflict. A settled opinion is the outcome of battling doubts and debates. Intense conflicts, if we are victorious, leave behind a sense of security and rest that it is scarcely possible to disturb again. And the storms and stress of youth lead to the tranquility of age. But all this is insufficient to justify the analogy, for by the principle of entropy no change at all should be possible when the state of equilibrium is reached ; and psycho-analysts believe that the unconscious can be very active. The only state of entropy would be the state of death when all doubts are quieted and all conflicts settled for ever as far as the individual is concerned.

Let us, now, see what modern physics make of the energy concept. The pre-relativity doctrine of energy considered it as something which had motive power ; in fact the sole source of motive power. Its measure was a mathematical function both of mass and velocity. No doubt for this reason it was adopted by psychologists in the attempt to make clear what the motive power of the mind really was like. Something in the nature of energy (in the popular sense of energetic) was required in order to explain the motive power of instinct and thought ; to construct, in fact, a dynamic psychology. No other physical concept, except one which contained the idea of ' power ' or ' efficacy ' would have served the purpose. Here was the concept of energy, lying ready to hand, with the necessary properties and accredited antecedents. As psychology has always hankered after becoming respectable by being considered as a natural science, it promptly adopted energy which appeared to have such good credentials in the matter of power or motive force.

Unfortunately, however, modern physics has deprived energy of all its activity, for it now identifies energy with mass (11) ; and regards causality as a symmetrical relation, and not as the one-way relation of cause and effect. Dynamics is being rapidly reduced to geometry, and Einstein's theory has converted gravitational force into a property of curved space. (12) The sun has no more ' power ' to pull the earth to itself than the hypotenuse of a right-angled triangle to attract the other two sides to its extremities. I am far from saying that this conception of causality ought to be applied to mental phenomena. But, as psychologists, we cannot have it both ways. If ideas are borrowed from physics we must take what physics offers, and the analogies employed must not give physical concepts implications which physicists themselves reject, or which are only true of bygone physical ideas. If energy has no ' power ' in the physical world what is the sense of employing its analogue in the mental realm for a dynamic psychology ? It is far better to desist from using the term mental energy and to confine ourselves to the notion of mental activity with which we have direct acquaintance. By the use of the above analogy nothing is explained, nothing is made clearer, and its employment merely serves to cloak our complete ignorance, and to hinder investigation. What is worse it makes us content with explanations which are palpably inadequate or definitely erroneous. And Dr E. D. Adrian surely summed up the position accurately when he said that there is no reason to suppose that " mental energy will follow any of the generalizations which have been observed for energy changes in material systems." (13) Our study of Jung's attempt to work out the analogy has fully justified this belief.

It is now time to turn to the experimental facts and other evidence in order to see how far they are consistent with the views expressed above. If the analogy of psycho-physical energy with material energy had any foundation in fact, it ought to be easy to shew a diminution of energy as the result of fatigue.　For fatigue would diminish the capacity to do work since the available energy would be used up.　The volume of research devoted to this subject is overwhelming and some attempt has been made in my *Educational Psychology* to get a conspectus of it and evaluate it. (14)　Most of the work has been devoted to the attempt to find evidence for the supposed diminution of energy after physical or mental labour.　The conclusions reached by the different investigators, using the same methods, have been mutually conflicting ; and the suspicion arises that what they have been looking for does not exist.　Incredible feats have been performed to display the diminution of capacity by the using up of the hypothetical energy.　Martyrs have sacrificed themselves on this altar in order to use up their store of energy ; but with no avail. For example, eight college students performed arithmetical additions for 10 hours on end ; and it was found that the average number of examples correctly done in the first and last 10 minute periods was 38.4 and 37.9 respectively.　The average number correct in the tenth minute of the day was 38 and in the last minute of all was 42. (15)　This affords no evidence whatever for the assumption of a fund or reserve of energy which is being drawn upon and diminished.

Our admiration for this effort would be boundless, were it not that it pales into insignificance in comparison with the heroic attempt of a Japanese student. (16)　If ever a person made a serious effort to drain her fund of mental energy this student did.　For four successive days, for 12 hours each day, she multiplied two four-figure numbers, *e.g.* 2645 × 5784 *in her head*, memorizing not only the processes but the numbers themselves, disdaining to have them written in front of her. There were no pauses on any of the days, except to record the time, not even for meals !　On every day she accomplished about 70 examples.　The time taken for each successive set of 10 examples increased on any day, whilst the average number of errors made in each successive set of 10 on the fourth day was:

Set	1	2	3	4	5	6	7
Errors	2.0	1.5	2.1	2.1	1.6	4.1	3.1

Professor E. L. Thorndike, in whose laboratory the work was done, is amply justified in his sober comment : " The amount of loss in absolute efficiency was probably very slight. For a person to be able to multiply a number like 9263 by one like 5748 without any visual, written, or spoken aids, even in fifteen, or for that matter in a hundred and fifty minutes, implies a very high degree of efficiency. That a person can exert himself to the utmost at this very difficult work for ten or twelve hours without rest and still able to do it, even at the expense of twice or thrice as many minutes per example as at the beginning, means that the loss in efficiency by any absolute standard has been small." (17). Results of a like kind, though of less heroic quality, are common in experimental investigations on fatigue. In fact if anybody were prepared to maintain that, *under suitably controlled conditions*, it has not been possible to discover *any* diminution of capacity for work, no matter how prolonged or difficult the task, no convincing experimental evidence could be brought to confute him.

General observation leads to the same conclusion. The amount of continuous wearing work which women perform for their loved ones or to alleviate distress is inconsistent with any theory based on a fund of energy. In pursuit of a cherished purpose their energy appears to be inexhaustible. A couple of examples may be cited in support of this assertion. The first is taken from Mr Lytton Strachey's *Eminent Victorians* and relates to the utterly incredible quantity of work performed by Florence Nightingale over a long series of years when she had become an invalid. At the age of thirty-seven, after two years in the Crimea under conditions calculated to kill the strongest constitution, she returned to England with a bad attack of fever. Her nervous system was undermined, her heart was affected, she suffered constantly from fainting fits and attacks of utter physical prostration. " The doctors declared that one thing alone would save her—a complete and prolonged rest. But that was the one thing with which she would have nothing to do. The doctors protested in vain ; in vain her family lamented and entreated. As she lay upon her sofa, gasping, she devoured blue-books, dictated letters and, in the intervals of her palpitations, cracked her febrile jokes. For months at a time she never left her bed. For years she was in daily expectation of death. But she would not rest. At this rate, the doctors assured her, even if she did not die, she would become an invalid for life. She could not help that ; there was the work to be done ", and she set about doing it.

In the teeth of the most determined opposition, after persistent labour, she forced the Government to appoint a commission for which she drew up a report that remains to this day the leading authority on the medical administration of armies. " Her health was almost desperate ; but she did not flinch, and after six months of incredible industry she had put together and written with her own hand her ' Notes affecting the health, efficiency, and hospital administration of the British Army '. This extraordinary composition filled more than eight hundred closely printed pages and contained an enormous mass of information—military, statistical, sanitary, and architectural ". She then spent another six months on the very brink of death perpetually working so as to secure the adoption of her recommendations. Year after year she carried on this feverish activity, more and more ravenous for work. She wrote a tract which revolutionized the theory of hospital construction and management, and founded a training school for nurses. The latter would have been enough to absorb the whole efforts of at least two lives of ordinary vigour but she simultaneously carried on an astonishing number of other activities. At the age of fifty she settled down with somewhat better health, but still an invalid " who was too weak to walk downstairs and who worked far harder than most Cabinet Ministers ". Besides her public work she wrote a philosophical-religious book in three large volumes and acted as occasional adviser to her own and foreign governments on difficult questions of army administration. For the best part of forty years she kept up this strenuous mode of existence and finally died at the age of ninety-one. Whoever can believe that the source of all this activity was a fund of energy in such a feeble human body must indeed be possessed of great and simple faith.

The second example is taken from Anthony Trollope's *Autobiography*, and refers to his mother's amazing exertions as an author in the face of overwhelming odds. (18) When she was well over fifty she began to write novels in order, by her unaided efforts to support a ruined, penniless family. Her husband, a son and daughter were dying from consumption and she carried on her literary efforts whilst nursing them. Every morning she rose at 4 o'clock and did her writing before anybody was awake. " My mother's most visible occupation was that of nursing. There were two sick men in the house and hers were the hands that tended them. The novels went on, of course. We had already learned to know that they would be forthcoming at stated intervals—and they were always forthcoming. The doctor's vials and the ink bottles held equal places in my mother's room. . . . My mother went through it unscathed in strength, though she performed all the work of the day nurse and night nurse to a sick household ; for there were soon three of them dying. . . . It was about this period of her career that her best novels were written ". Subsequently she established a home for her daughter and another for herself by her unaided efforts. But this did not exhaust her energy, for she continued writing vigorously till she was 76 years old " and had at that time produced 114 volumes of which the first was not written till she was fifty." Trollope's remark, that her career offers great encouragement " to those who have not begun early to do something before they depart hence," appears mildly and unnecessarily laconic. These examples seem almost to have been invented in order to make the theory of a fund of energy appear startlingly paradoxical. It seems to me that instances of this kind, which could be multiplied, are convincing evidence that spiritual energy is *toto coelo* different from any form of physical energy. In the accomplishment of a cherished purpose we have no warrant for assuming that spiritual energy is exhaustible. The sum of human " energy " is capable of indefinite increase in the service of any noble ideal. We have not only to revise our psychological concepts, but to remember that in the realm of ideals any attempt to equate the physical with the spiritual view of energy is to shut our eyes to the most obvious facts around us.

William James was too good a student of human nature to be oblivious of such facts as I have given, and he wrote a famous essay with the title " *The Energies of Men* " in which he called attention to similar observations. He wrote as follows : " The words ' energy ' and ' maximum ' may easily suggest only quantity to the reader's mind, whereas in measuring human energies, qualities as well as quantities have to be taken into account. Every one feels that his total *power* rises when he passes to a higher *qualitative* level " (his italics). Of course he does. But it is bad logic and worse psychology to convert this vivid but highly metaphorical description of levels into a quantitative reality ; though James went dangerously near to such a metamorphosis in the delightful essay just quoted. Still, he never quite meant what he said, and he would, in all probability, have been greatly puzzled to learn that his metaphorical *qualitative* levels could by some miraculous agency be converted to a single quantitative fund of energy. What impressed James was the complete absence of any signs of diminished vitality where complete exhaustion of ' energy ' might have been expected. He endeavoured to explain this phenomenon by the phrase ' qualitative levels ', a happy rhetorical expression devoid of any meaning ; for how can *levels* be qualitative ?

Professor C. Spearman, strangely enough, calls James to witness in support of his views. (19) He maintains that the concept of mental energy is based primarily on what he calls the constancy of mental output, but " a further and hardly less powerful reason has been found in the phenomena that fall under the heading of fatigue ". What these phenomena are he does not indicate ; nor where the experimental or other evidence for them can be found, though he refers to James, McDougall and Janet, none of whom provides it. He is obviously under the impression that somebody or other has, at some time, been able to measure mental fatigue and to shew that its essential ' phenomenon ' consists of a diminution in mental output. On any other assumption the existence of mental fatigue can give no such support to the doctrine of mental energy as the theory requires. I believe that a totally different explantion of mental fatigue can be given, which is consistent with all the experimental evidence and has the additional advantage of accounting for the qualitative facts considered above.

Before giving this explanation it will be as well to sum up the argument to this point. The idea currently held of mental fatigue, and supported by eminent psychologists, rests on the doctrine of mental energy, whereby it is supposed that each person has at his disposal a definite fund of such energy. This concept was borrowed from physics, as it seemed to have the two properties necessary for a psychological explanation ; namely constancy in quantity and efficiency or ' power '. Consequently the concept has been used to lend support to certain theories of the unconscious, instinct and intelligence. But the modern doctrine of energy assigns to its properties which are totally different from those demanded by most psychologists, for the physicist's energy is simply a mathematical abstraction. Dr Jung sees this clearly and for him libido is merely an expression for the energic standpoint. He says " The libido with which we work is not only not concrete or recognizable, but is a complete X, a pure hypothesis, a picture or a counter, which is just as little concretely conceived as is the energy of the world known to physics ". The point of the analogy, therefore, breaks down. Appeal is also made to experiments on fatigue. Researches on fatigue make use of the doctrine since the researchers have assumed that theoretical psychology has established it as a tenable hypothesis ; whereas theoretical psychology employs the hypothesis under the impression that the doctrine has been established by researches on fatigue. So the wheel has come full circle. Is it too sanguine to hope that during its revolution it may have whizzed off the theory of a fund of mental energy ?

If we cannot measure mental fatigue by the diminution of a hypothetical fund of psycho-physical energy how are we to proceed ? For fatigue is undoubtedly something real, and must have measurable properties. I have endeavoured to shew elsewhere that the experimental evidence may be interpreted as an interference with steady or rhythmical vital activity. (14) This is the essential phenomenon of fatigue, the effect of which is not necessarily to diminish the amount we are able to do ; it may even increase it, owing, probably, to the stimulation of the nerves by poisonous metabolites. In a state of fatigue a person loses control of his voluntary activity ; he becomes unsteady and wavering and is unable to exercise that steady rhythmical control which is necessary to the production of good work. Hence the industrial psychologists have been wise in attempting to measure fatigue by the amount of spoilt work or the number of accidents ; since both of these are indications of a lack of controlled voluntary attention.

Professor E. L. Thorndike has also come to a similar conclusion. (17) He says " All the facts, both of experimental studies and of everyday life support the hypothesis that the effects of continuous exercise upon *readiness* is far quicker, greater and more significant than its effect upon *maximum power*. Fatigue in the vague popular sense means that we are less willing rather than that we are less able, that the probability of achievement is decreased by the increased effort that it requires rather than that the possibility of achievement is decreased inevitably." This seems to me an admirable summary of what experimental facts and general observation have shewn, when the data are dispassionately examined, apart from any preconceived theory. The facts supplied by physiology also support this view. Thus Professor Sherrington (20) has shewn that the scratching reflex, produced by various stimuli, has a certain constancy of rhythm ; " under all these various modes of excitation (heat-beam, constant current, double and single induced currents, high frequency currents, and mechanical stimuli) the rhythm of the flexor response remains . . . almost the same ". When fatigue sets in owing to prolonged excitation the action becomes less steady and less accurately adjusted, " it becomes tremulous and the tremor becomes progressively more marked and irregular." The physiological explanation of this phenomenon has been given by Pavlov (21) in his work on conditioned reflexes. When a positive conditioned reflex is stimulated at a point on the skin then neighbouring areas on the skin act as inhibitors. And when a negative conditioned reflex is stimulated surrounding points become excitors. There is, in fact, a mutual induction of inhibition by excitation and *vice versa*. When there is a regular alternation of positive and inhibiting stimuli the reflexes are much more precise, since each phase assists the succeeding one. Hence rhythmic activity is performed more easily and with less exhaustion than arythmic activity. This is the physiological ground for the explanation of fatigue. It is not a question of quantity of activity but of rhythmical activity.

In order to test this conception of fatigue by further psychological experiment the following investigation was undertaken. Eight graduate students acted as subjects of the experiment, which was conducted in the evening. They were given a series of texts containing interesting historical matter, printed with no divisions between the words or paragraphs, no punctuation marks or capital letters ; the texts presenting the appearance of a continuous collection of letters. Their task was to divide the words by drawing short vertical lines between them and to indicate the full stops by making crosses. Marks were assigned for correct division of words and punctuation, and subtracted for errors. (22) The subjects worked continuously at this task for half an hour without any break ; and at the end of that time all declared that, though the work was interesting, they were tired out. This feeling of tiredness was both physical and mental, the former being due mainly to eye strain of which most of the subjects complained.

The table here given shews the median marks of the group for each of the thirty minutes.

Time	.	1	2	3	4	5	6	7	8	9	10
Marks	.	38	34	48	45	44	54	51	52	46	47
Time	.	11	12	13	14	15	16	17	18	19	20
Marks	.	48	49	51	53	54	56	51	49	51	47
Time	.	21	22	23	24	25	26	27	28	29	30
Marks	.	56	53	53	47	50	59	50	55	52	60

It will be seen that the marks shew a tendency to rise for the first 16 minutes, after which they hover round a more or less fixed centre. The coefficient or variation of the marks for each subject, for every consecutive five-minute period was calculated. This coefficient measures the regularity or *steadiness* with which the subjects are accomplishing their task within the period stated. The mean of such coefficients for the eight subjects for each of the successive periods was

1	2	3	4	5	6
13.8	6.6	7.7	7.3	9.6	9.5

At first the coefficient is high, as the subjects have not yet adjusted themselves to the task, and are consequently very irregular in their performance. In the next five minutes adjustment has been secured and the big drop in the coefficient shews that the work is being steadily pursued. For the next ten minutes the work is still steady but less so than in the previous period. During the last ten minutes the coefficients shew that the work is being very irregularly performed ; whilst the former table indicates that the amount of work accomplished during this period shews no tendency to decrease. By analogy with the experiments of other observers given above, it is reasonable to assume that if the task had been continued for several hours there would be no diminution in the quantity of work done for each period. It is evident that there is no reason to assume that a fund of energy is being used up, but that the phenomenon of fatigue is displayed in the greater irregularity of the activity employed. Fatigue militates against steadiness, owing to the lack of control of voluntary attention. In the experiments previously quoted in which eight college students performed arithmetical additions for 10 hours, the coefficients of variability for the first and last 10 minute periods were 6.7 and 8.7 respectively, an increase of thirty per cent. ; though there was no diminution in quantity.

Further evidence tending in the same direction has been supplied by the carefully timed record of an athlete while covering 200 yards at top speed. (23) Accurate timing was made by a series of coils at equal distances above the track and connected to a galvanometer. The runner carried a thin flexible magnetized steel ribbon round his waist. Each time he passed a coil the magnet induced a current which was recorded photographically. The following table shews the time at which he passed each 20 yard mark. In the third line I have indicated the time for covering each distance, in the fourth the coefficient of variability. As the runner did not settle down to a steady pace until he had passed the first 20 yard mark the calculations of the coefficients start from that point. It is a pity that the coils were not placed at intervals of 10 or 5 yards, when the theory could have been more adequately tested. The results, however, shew an increased variability with distance, and thus confirm the previous data in an unexpected manner.

Distance (yds.)	20	40	60	80	100	120	140
Time (secs.)	2.760	4.595	6.380	8.125	9.885	11.695	13.550
Time (per 20 yds.)	2.760	1.835	1.785	1.745	1.760	1.810	1.855

Coefficient of Variability   1.73   1.79

Distance (yds.)	160	180	200
Time (secs.)	15.455	17.425	19.455
Time (per 20 yds.)	1.905	1.970	2.030

Coefficient of Variability   2.15

The conclusions forced on us by the facts of everyday life and experimental investigation thus confirm each other. Where the doctrine of a fund of energy can be brought to the test it breaks down completely. We have found it possible to give an explanation of fatigue which ignores the hypothesis ; and the results of experiment support the explanation. Just as physiologists have found it is advisable to give up the idea of nervous energy, and employ that of nervous activity instead, so for psychological purposes we are forced to abandon the conception. Vital activity, physical or mental, is rhythmical and as long as a person is fresh the rhythm is sustained and regular ; but with prolonged activity it becomes more and more difficult to maintain the regular swing of action, which finally breaks down. The subjective impression of this lack of steadiness is what we call the feeling of fatigue and is a warning to us to desist. Anything which helps the rhythm tends to ward off this feeling, as is well shewn by the fact that soldiers can march longer and more easily to the strains of music ; and all bodily labour is made less fatiguing by rhythmical action.

In experimental investigations and in everyday life where a diminution of capacity has been observed as a consequence of prolonged activity the result is a secondary phenomenon. Inability to control attention may, of course, express itself in a diminished output of work but, as we have abundantly seen, this is by no means an inevitable or necessary occurrence. Other phenomena are much more certain and primary. Such are errors, accidents, spoilt work, a tired feeling and all the other results of an uncontrolled and wavering attention. It is to these that we must look as the surest indicators of fatigue and not to some purely imaginary store of energy which has no warrant in theory or in practice.

The conclusion of the whole matter is this. When we speak of mental activity we are using a term whose connotation is known to us by immediate experience. We have a direct acquaintance with activity in ourselves whenever we make an effort to think. In fact it is certain that when we speak of the activity of inanimate things we do so by a translation into them of something which we know directly only in our own consciousness. Here the analogy is from the mental to the physical realm. But the direction is reversed when we make use of such expressions as a narrow minded man or a man of wide outlook or a person whose ideas run in a groove. All these and the like expressions convey something perfectly definite which we can only characterize by means of analogies taken from material objects. Their use is justified by the limitations of our vocabulary and the consequent tendency to find analogies to illustrate our meaning. So it is reasonable to speak of the mind expanding as the result of education, and indeed it would be difficult and tedious to express what we mean in any other terminology. But it would be idle to suppose that the analogy can be pushed further and that the laws of expansion of gases (say) apply to the expansion of the mind. When we increase the pressure of instruction we may decrease the volume of what is learnt, but only a very fanciful psychologist could imagine that, therefore, we are justified in applying Boyle's law to mental development. Similarly it is necessary sometimes to refer to the mind's elasticity but there is no reason whatever to suppose that Hooke's law applies to this characteristic of mind. The use of the concept of mental energy as a descriptive analogical term may be allowed on the ground of poverty of language and convenience ; but to assume that the quantitative laws of physical energy apply to the mental sphere, or that there is a fund of mental energy, is to exceed the bounds of legitimate scientific procedure.

CHAPTER VIII

INSTINCT AND CUSTOM

IF there is one thing more than another in psychology which seems to cry aloud for both mental energy and a fixed nervous structure it is the doctrine of instinct. As we have thrown doubt on both these concepts it is our obvious duty to tackle the problem of instincts in human activity. Locke had compared the mind, at the outset of its experience, to an empty cabinet or a ' white paper, void of all characters '. The mind had simply certain general capacities, such as memory, just as a sheet of paper has the property of retaining marks made upon it. And just as a sheet of paper has no preference for any particular writing so the mind has no inclination in any specific direction. Leibniz, in opposition to this view, had compared the mind to a block of marble which was not homogeneous but had certain veins in it. From a homogeneous block a sculptor could carve any figure indifferently, but from a veined block one particular form in preference to others would be easier to obtain ; just as Michael Angelo is said to have given the awkward position of the dropped shoulder in his David as a result of the curious elongated shape of the block of marble from which he chiselled it. In this sense Leibniz held that one particular figure in preference to others would be in some way innate in the marble ; though, of course, it would still be necessary for the genius of the artist to produce the figure by working in the way determined by the marble. " Thus ideas and truths are innate as inclinations, dispositions, habitudes or possibilities which may become actualities ".

Leaving aside ideas and truths as belonging to the province of philosophy, and discarding material analogies, what the psychology of instinct has to discuss is whether dispositions, inclinations, etc., can, in any intelligible sense, be said to be inborn in the mind. In order to investigate this it is obviously necessary to have some criterion by which we can determine whether a particular tendency is inborn or acquired. The mere fact of a disposition appearing late or early in the life history of an individual cannot be used as a criterion, since it is perfectly possible for an impulse to mature late though it is an original part of human nature.

William James believed that the inexplicable and psychologically obvious character of any impulse, and the satisfaction derived from acting in accordance with it, were sound reasons for believing in its originality. Neither natural selection nor the pleasure derived from pursuing certain aims was capable of explaining inborn impulses. (1) "Why," he asks, "do various animals do what seem to us such strange things in the presence of such outlandish stimuli ? Why does the hen, for example, submit herself to the tedium of incubating such a fearfully uninteresting set of objects as a nestful of eggs ? Why do men always lie down, when they can on soft beds rather than on hard floors ? . . . Why do they prefer saddle of mutton and champagne to hard-tack and ditch water ? Why does the maiden interest the youth so that everything about her seems more important and significant than anything else in the world ? Nothing more can be said than that these are human ways, and that every creature *likes* its own ways, and takes to following them as a matter of course. . . . It takes what Berkeley called a mind debauched by learning to carry the process of making the natural seem strange, so far as to ask for the *why* of any instinctive human act." Other criteria have been employed to distinguish instinctive from acquired impulses, in addition to their non-rationality and satisfyingness. One of the chief of these is the feeling or interest which is at the kernel of an instinct ; the feeling, so to speak, that the action prompted by the instinctive impulse is worth while. Another is that every instinct is liable to perversion in some individuals. But, of course, this must be strictly limited, since if the majority of individuals acted in a perverse way the latter mode would be instinctive. Thus, some mothers are cruel to their children, but if the great

M

majority of mothers were so, then cruelty would be the maternal instinct. Again, the ineradicability of an impulse is regarded as a sure sign that the disposition is part of the original nature of man. For what cannot be rooted out of the constitution must be part of the native endowment of the mind.

Using the criteria of ultimate inexplicability and originality, and basing himself on the observations of earlier writers, James gave an inventory of man's original equipment. This includes such sensation-reflexes as sucking, clasping, carrying things to the mouth, vocalization ; and then proceeds to such motor activities as sitting up, standing, walking. Instinctive activities as pugnacity, hunting, fear reactions, the parental instinct, gregariousness, curiosity, acquisitiveness are enumerated. Complex tendencies, as preference for sheltered places, play, love of ceremony, etc., are all part of the native endowment of the mind. And in addition several emotions such as envy, resentment, jealousy, modesty are included. For James believed that " every object that excites an instinct excites an emotion as well. The only distinction that one may draw is that the reaction called emotional terminates in the subject's own body, whilst the reaction called instinctive is apt to go further and enter into practical relations with the exciting object."

Now it is patent that, if this curious and miscellaneous assortment of tendencies to action are inborn, the above list is by no means complete, but is merely a sample. Accordingly Professor E. L. Thorndike (2), although he does not pretend to be complete, devotes eight chapters of his *Educational Psychology* to an enumeration of unlearned tendencies or original nature in man. He begins with reflexes and sensation-reflexes, bodily control, and proceeds to such complex activities as pugnacity, hunting, collecting and hoarding, etc., and enumerates several emotional tendencies such as fear, pugnacity, anger, etc. In addition he enumerates a group of tendencies which are responses to the behaviour of other people, such as imitation, gregariousness, motherly behaviour, paternal instinct, masterly and submissive behaviour, rivalry, sex behaviour during courtship, etc. Such responses as teasing, bullying, envy and jealousy, etc., are also included, and a variety of other simple or complicated reactions to various social or non-social situations. The above are, of course, but samples of his list and he does not pretend to be complete ; so various and extensive are the elements included in the original nature of man.

One of the great services rendered to the study of the mind by Professor McDougall was to emphasize the functional aspect of mental dispositions, and thereby to provide psychologists with a sharply defined concept of instinct in place of the hazy and shifting idea previously held. His definition of an instinct, which has the merit of being approved by Dr J. Drever (3) who has made a special study of instinct in man, is as follows (4) : " an innate disposition which determines its possessor to perceive (pay attention to) any object of a certain class, and to experience in its presence a certain emotional excitement and an impulse to action which find expression in a specific mode of behaviour in relation to that object ". The inborn disposition is compared to a lock and the object to a key which unlocks it ; and just as each type of lock can only be opened by a particular sort of key, so each instinct can only be aroused by a particular class of objects. By the use of the criteria set out in the above definition McDougall enumerates " all the instincts that seem to me to be comprised in the innate constitution of the human species." Apart from certain minor instincts there are thirteen of these, namely : the parental instinct, the combative, curiosity, the instinct of escape, the food seeking instinct, disgust, the herd instinct, self-assertion and its opposite, the sexual instinct, the acquisitive, the constructive, and the instinct of appeal. All these are ineradicable parts of the structure of the mind, and experience can only modify their action but cannot change their nature. Professor McDougall teaches, and I think correctly, that an instinctive disposition must be specific, otherwise there is nothing that could be called instinctive in it ; but he is careful to point out that the specificity of instincts both on the receptive and executive sides is of very different degrees. Moreover, it would be generally agreed that unless the disposition were common to the whole species there is nothing in it which could be rightly regarded as instinctive.

In opposition to all this, the thesis I propose to maintain in this chapter is that the concept of instinct is inapplicable to human activity, however useful it may be in explaining the actions of lower animals, especially invertebrates. Our study of the nervous system has shewn that there is no reason to suppose that there are ready formed mechanisms which predispose to particular lines of activity ; but rather that all parts of the central nervous system are functionally inter-changeable. Further, the study of human instinct is not concerned with the physiology of instinctive mechanisms but, as Dr J. Drever has so persuasively maintained, with mental predispositions. And McDougall's definition is entirely couched in mental terms. This was the point of view which Samuel Butler very forcibly presented in his work on *Life and Habit*, and which has never been seriously challenged. Now a functional disposition without some activity and an environ-ment, which gives it form, is an empty conception, or rather a meaningless one. Despite poetic sanction to the contrary there is no meaning in talking of a " mute inglorious Milton ". Unless a man has composed poetry there is no sense whatever in regarding him as a poet, however good a ploughman he is. A naked possibility is nothing ; or as Leibniz remarked a *puissance ou faculté nue* is an absurdity. If this were not the case, there would be nothing to smile at in the reply of the man, who, on being asked whether he played the violin, answered that he did not know because he had never tried.

If there were no keys in the world there could be no locks. Here the danger of using non-biological analogies in psychology is peculiarly evident. For it is supposed to be quite easy to see how a lock could exist without there being any keys whereas, as a matter of fact, the idea of a lock would be meaningless in that case. The only thing that would exist would be pieces of curiously shaped metal ; not a lock. Similarly an organism apart from its environment is a meaning-less abstraction. And, coming nearer to our subject matter, we may likewise say that an instinct without some corresponding specific features in the biological or social environment is an empty or meaningless conception. If then it can be shewn that so-called instinctive human activity is invariably dependent on some particular social environment, there would seem to be no room for separate independent instincts. Now I maintain that this can be shewn in the case of every activity which is denominated instinctive. By universal consent the strongest instincts in human beings are the sexual and the maternal and parental instincts ; for which reason I shall illustrate my remarks mainly from these. As these springs of action have well-defined physiological organs it may reasonably be assumed that if instinct is to be sought for anywhere in human life they must be found here.

If there were a true parental instinct there could be no distinction in respect of parental behaviour between sons and daughters. Yet there are certain peoples amongst whom daughters are disregarded, and parental affection is lavished on the sons. C. M. Doughty (5) who lived among the Beduin for a long time, as one of themselves, thus describes their difference of attitude. " Daughters when past the first amiable infancy are little set by in Arabic households. The son is beloved by his father, till he be grown, above the wife that bare him, before his own soul, and next after the man's own father : and the young child [*i.e.* boy] in an household is hardly less beloved of his elder brethren. God has sent a son, and the father cannot contrary him in anything, whilst he is a child. This it is that in time to come may comfort his age, and in his last end honourably bury him ; and the year by year after, as the nomads in their journeys be come again, offer the sacrifices of the dead and pray over him ; so shall his name be yet had in remembrance among the living. . . . A son dying, a father's spirit is long overcast, he is overborne awhile with silent sorrow ; but the remembrance of a deceased daughter, unless her life were of any singular worth or goodly promise untimely broken, is not very long enduring." I suppose we get nearer to unsophisticated human nature when dealing with Beduin than with Western Europeans.

It is clear from the above that parental behaviour to off-spring is entirely a matter of social custom. And anybody who is familiar with the unintentional cruelty of English parents to their children in the early decades of the nineteenth century in the cause of their education can easily convince himself of this. Flogging, starvation and other methods of bending the will to virtue were employed and approved in the interests of the children's welfare ; and parental instinct was submerged in the social atmosphere of the time. If the course of action pursued is entirely a matter of social custom what is the use of speaking of instincts ? It is perhaps worth remarking, what has often been pointed out before, that the moral worth of a particular action or mode of conduct is entirely independent of the fact whether it is inborn or acquired. Parental action is just as admirable or reprehensible if it is acquired.

Perhaps it may be urged that, at any rate, maternal behaviour is due to an instinct. Here the matter is equally difficult to decide since in every stage of civilization the rearing of children is so much a family or tribal concern, and no woman is left alone to act for herself. Professor J. B. Watson (6) describes what happens in maternity wards, where the usual social conventions and customs are largely replaced by others. After quoting how maternal instincts are usually described he goes on to say. " To those who work in maternity wards the situation is sometimes seen to be quite otherwise. We have observed the nursing, handling, bathing, etc. of the first baby of a good many mothers. Certainly there are no new ready-made activities appearing except nursing. The mother is usually as awkward about that as she can well be. The instinctive factors are practically *nil*. The emotional activity of both parents may be intense, but this is often the result of many factors. Very often the mother who is unshackled by social conventions behaves quite differently. Even in cases where the woman is duly married and there is no reason for a transfer of an emotional state of an adverse kind upon the child, little maternal behaviour of the type usually described appears. *Society puts the strongest pressure upon a conventional attitude with respect to the proper care of*

*the youngster and the emotional attitude which should be displayed
with reference to it* (italics mine). We are not denying however
that there are some instinctive factors here. It should be
recalled that the nursing of the child and the fondling of it
is not without a sex stimulating effect upon the mother. . . .
Just to the extent to which convention permits it, rationaliza-
tion [of maternal conduct] occurs. This is a strong argument
that maternal behaviour is not mainly instinctive." But, of
course, it is none the less admirable.

The practice of infanticide again seems to establish the fact
that parental conduct is entirely determined by social convention. In sharp contrast to the modern anxiety to lessen
child mortality there is sound historical evidence, backed up
by the direct observation of the behaviour of primitive groups
in modern times, that this practice was widespread. Among
the various groups of primitive folk of Tasmania and Australia
infanticide was common, and was also practised widely among
hunting races as the Eskimos. (7) Certain agricultural races
in North and especially South America had this custom and
in some cases the first child, if a girl, was always killed. The
custom was very prevalent amongst the New Zealanders and
in Polynesia. A famous secret society in the Society Islands
enjoined the killing of all children on its members by oath.
The first missionaries published it as their opinion that in the
Islands as a whole not less than two-thirds of the children
were murdered by their own parents. The natives of Mada-
gascar and the Hottentots also practised infanticide.

Passing to civilized peoples we find exactly the same state
of affairs. In historical times in Greece the practice is said
to have been universal, and the murder was usually ordered
by the father, the child being exposed and left to die. In the
ideal legislature of Plato and Aristotle the practice was
enjoined, as it was also by the practical legislation of Lycurgus
and Solon. Glotz who has examined all the evidence thus
sums it up " L'opinion de la Grèce ancienne est donc a peu
près unanime. Reçue dans la vie privée, cette pratique a été
admise en droit par les législatures et fondée en raison par
les maîtres de la pensée." Infanticide was general in Rome

in very early times, but the father's rights were somewhat restricted later. Many women exposed their children and the custom was regarded as quite natural. Thus in the Golden Ass of Apuleius a husband before going on a journey directed his young wife that the coming babe, if a girl, was to be destroyed, and this is related as a perfectly natural and common occurrence. It was also very prevalent among the Arabs before Mohammed forbade it. In China and India the custom was common until the last generation and no criminality was attached to infanticide. It was estimated that in 1874 more than one-half of the girls born in Rajputana were destroyed. And before their conversion to Christianity the custom was extensively practised amongst the Teutonic tribes.

Moreover as Professor A. M. Carr-Saunders (8) has pointed out there has often been a bias on the part of observers to disregard evidence about infanticide and similar practices. " Many observers are attracted by the races who come under their notice and seem to think that these practices are incompatible with the kindly nature or pleasant disposition of the people they describe—that in fact the attribution to them of such customs as a normal feature of existence is a kind of libel—and if they report them at all, they persuade themselves into thinking that they are infrequent and abnormal. We have only to remember the objection taken to the interpretation of the finds in neoloithic graves in England as evidences of infanticide—an objection based on the dislike of believing that our ancestors could have been guilty of such a habit—or, again, we may remember that Tacitus, when desirous of holding up the Germanic tribes as an example to the Romans of his day, declared that they never committed infanticide— the implication being that infanticide is to be regarded as a degenerate and unworthy custom. Nevertheless in spite of the bias against belief there is ample evidence that one or more of these practices are recorded for almost every people."

If the practice is thus nearly universal then either the parental instinct is non-existent or too weak to overcome the most repulsive actions contrary to it ; or else we are almost driven to the belief that, for the human species, infanticide and similar practices are instinctive. What is the sense of referring certain human activities to instinctive tendencies when peoples in all ages and climes have not acted in accordance with them ? Rather we are forced to the conclusion that custom hardened into habit is the great motive force of human action.

An exactly similar state of affairs to that described above prevails with regard to the sexual instinct, which plays so prominent a part in modern psychological discussions, especially of a popular kind. In this matter sociologists and ethnologists have much to teach us. There is a widespread belief that the manifestations of the sexual instinct are so ' natural ' that society should have no more concern about it, except in so far as it leads to procreation, than it should over the food we eat, or the manifestations of any other appetite. Dr C. W. Margold (9) has shewn that the assumed distinction between social and individual sex conduct is unsound. The biological point of view is never adequate to account for human conduct, for the social medium in which a person lives is not something antithetical to his personality but an essential factor in it. " The theoretical conception of a sexual life existing apart from control, more or less effective, by the public opinion of the community, is unreal, incompatible with human nature, never realized." It is an abstraction to regard sexual conduct, or any other conduct for the matter of that, as something individually generated from the biologically given. Any account of human conduct that regards our physiological organism as the determiner of our acts ignores the essential factor of what is socially given.

It is an obvious corollary that all human impulses are so infinitely plastic that they may be organized into any disposition, and have so been organized from time to time. What particular activities shall ensue are never determined by inborn impulses alone, for these are blind or indeterminate. And, as far as human action is concerned, biological equipment and social heritage are mutually involved and the latter is always the guiding factor. Human nature is not something predetermined by the organism and embodied in organs, but something in its very essence social ; found only in communities. We may confidently affirm, therefore, that no act can be predicted from a man's biological constitution, but that the content and form of every human activity is essentially social.

Accordingly as Dr Margold (10) has demonstrated, by an examination of the peoples where sexual promiscuity is tolerated and premarital chastity unknown, there is clear evidence even here of the invariable presence of social factors. These take the form of particular taboos or group ideals or social controls of various kinds, which may appear to us ridiculous, but are nevertheless potent. Thus among the Trobriands as studied by B. Malinowski, while a girl's father may have sexual relations with her, brothers and sisters are kept stringently apart not only in sexual intercourse but in what we might consider ordinary friendly relations. " Indeed, a Trobriand Islander, deeming physical resemblance somehow a sign of sexual intimacy, will consider it an outrageous insult and especially degrading to be told that he in the slightest degree resembles his sister."

If these observations are sound, even in cases where there is sexual promiscuity, then it is obvious that social control over private conduct should be more evident in other cases. And the study of ethnology bears this out. Accordingly we find the greatest possible diversity in sex practices from people to people. In fact sex behaviour, so far from being the direct result of a natural instinct is probably the most diverse of all behaviour of human beings. Every element in it is prescribed, ordered and regulated by the customs of the particular group. Thus kissing is or was unknown to a large number of races ; and a Burmese lover, for instance, does not kiss but smells the cheek of his mistress, whilst Maori lovers used to press their noses sideways. And the modes of courtship are almost as various as the numbers of different peoples. It is reported that among the Garos of Assam a girl considers herself insulted if her sweetheart speaks to her first about getting married. The age at which boys or girls may marry is determined entirely by the particular social group in which they happen to be born ; as we see in modern India. Moreover it is a commonplace amongst anthropologists that physical attractiveness in girls or boys is largely determined by fashion. It is not so long since the wearing of a bustle was an attempt to live up to the social idea of what constituted female beauty in civilized races. Amongst some peoples no woman will consider a man beautiful unless he has blackened his teeth. Females of the Sitka Islands cut their lower lip at the time of puberty, and gradually enlarge it so that they eventually look frightful to our eyes, but the natives consider it a mark of the highest beauty and try to make it as large as possible. Strange as it may appear to us, even the parts of the body which are supposed to be sexually attractive vary from group to group. Thus Mahommedan women, who were brought up to veil their faces in public, are said to have blushed if seen by men with the face uncovered. And it is reported that if chanced upon by strange men, whilst bathing, they were concerned only about covering the face. The practically nude natives of Sumatra and Celebes carefully cover the knee and consider it most improper to expose it, according to Westermarck. It is only a few years since European women have been allowed to expose their ankles or calves. And Indian women of the Caribbees transgress the rules of decency if they go out without being painted ; the two inch covering that they wear being regarded as less important in this respect.

Thus it is in accordance with the facts to say that (10) " No matter how odd, even how handicapping, immoral or positively reprehensible, from our own group notions, group sex practices may be, if individuals are from childhood brought up in them, if they see them valued, approved and practised in close and intimate association, if they are taught them as right, proper and decent, they will also invariably practise, approve and value them."

If more evidence is required of the essentially social and customary nature of sex behaviour it is abundantly furnished by observing the customs of the Japanese. Amongst them young men and women do not meet socially and no friendship is possible. They do not court one another. All the amenities of Western civilization such as dancing, mixed parties, dramatics are unknown. Marriage is entirely a family concern and social relationships between the sexes before marriage is not a necessary preliminary. A Japanese despises alike romance and sentimentality and marriage is regarded not as a purely private or personal matter but essentially a social concern. Of course sexual appetite exists among them as amongst us, but it is not idealized and such passion is regarded as an emotion unworthy of a civilized race.

Mr G. C. Allen, who has spent many years in intimate association with the Japanese, puts the situation very clearly. (11) " Let us try," he says, " to put the whole matter from the standpoint of a normal Japanese. In Anglo-Saxon countries, he would say, the sex relationship is idealized to an absurd extent, and love between the sexes is exaggerated into one of the greatest experiences of life. Western poetry, novels, and popular tradition serve to elevate what is merely a form of mutual hypnotism into the end-all and be-all of existence . . . what is in essence merely a trick of nature for securing the continuance of the species is held on occasion a justification for disloyalty and ingratitude. When two people feel drawn to one another, they are held to be justified in entering into a relationship which will have profound social consequences, and which will determine the future quality of the race. Any attempt which society may venture to make to control this relationship is resented as an infringement on liberty, and, curiously enough, as an unwarranted interference with a purely personal matter. These beliefs are so ingrained that they are the assumptions underlying most of the modern discussions of sex relationships. Yet English-speaking peoples conveniently ignore the fact that these ideas are common only to an insignificant proportion of the world's population, and that it is only within the last few centuries that they have come to form the basis of Western social philosophy."

Nor is it necessary to go to the Japanese to be convinced that there is no sex-instinct. In the next generation it will be difficult to get examples, for when Japanese and Chinese customs are completely assimilated to the European, psychologists will regard European customs as instinctive owing to their universality. Sexual behaviour, like all other behaviour, has to be learnt even though there is an appetite for this particular activity. Mr Bertrand Russell who is well aware of this, by a feat of mathematical logic, uses it as an argument for allowing absolute freedom in sexual conduct. His remarks on this matter of instinct are so pertinent, however, that I quote them. (12) " The instinctive element in sex relations is much less than is usually supposed. . . . The fact is that, where human beings are concerned, instinct is extraordinarily vague and easily turned aside from its natural course. The word ' instinct ', in fact, is hardly the proper one to apply to anything so far from rigid as human behaviour in sexual matters. I do not know how it may be with savages, but civilized people have to learn to perform the sexual act. It is not uncommon for doctors to be asked by married couples of some years' standing for advice as to how to get children, and to find on examination that the couples have not known how to perform intercourse. The sexual act is not, therefore, in the strictest sense instinctive, although of course there is a natural trend towards it ". If, then, there is no reason to believe that, for acts that have definite organs, there is an instinctive capacity to use them, it seems hard to believe that there are other instincts in human beings beyond those we have considered. Nevertheless the importance of the subject justifies some reference to these others.

Practically every list of human instincts contains the instinct of curiosity. As to this instinct, in the light of what has been said about the environment being an essential part of the function, it would be hard to demonstrate that all environments have sufficiently similar characters to render the meaning of such an instinct sufficiently definite to be worth considering. An instinct of curiosity, in the abstract, would appear to be devoid of meaning. Anybody who has read Doughty's *Travels in Arabia Deserta* can easily convince himself that the Beduin do not understand intellectual curiosity. They could not understand why anybody should want to come to Arabia and supposed that he must be seeking for treasure. His copying of inscriptions seemed to them a fatuous proceeding. On one occasion " East of Ybba Moghrair, we passed the foot of a little antique rude turret in the desert soil. I showed it to some riding next me in the rahla. ' Works (they answered) remaining from the creation of the world ; what profit is there to inquire of them ? ' " All that can be profitably said about curiosity is that in different places and at different times different peoples have been interested in different things, as the result of custom and tradition. With regard to such things they are curious, but absolutely ignore other things more interesting still. So little curious about the structure of the human body were the physicians of Europe that until the sixteenth century they were content to accept what the Greeks had taught without investigating for themselves. Macaulay was one of the best informed men concerning the literature and culture of ancient and modern Europe. But so little curious was he about Indian culture and traditions that, when he resided in India and drew up a scheme for Indian education, he brushed the whole of their literature and traditions aside as not worthy of consideration in a system of education. Similar examples could be multiplied indefinitely.

Those who provide lists of human instincts always include the tendency to collect and hoard, known as the acquisitive instinct. Now this is a topic that can be and has been investigated. Miss C. F. Burk (13) in the year 1900 examined over 600 boys and the same number of girls with regard to the collections they made. She found that only ten per cent. of boys and nine per cent. of girls were not actually making collections. The tendency was found to be the strongest at about the age of eleven or twelve but continued to adolescence, when it began to wane. This seemed to be very strong evidence of the existence of a hoarding instinct, and the investigation has been widely quoted since. In the year 1927 another inquiry was made in America, where they do these things on a statistical scale. (14) This time 5000 pupils of ages ranging from 9 to 22 years were investigated with reference to various kinds of collections, such as stamps, birds' eggs and so on. In contrast with the earlier enquiry it was found that the percentage of pupils making collections of one sort or another was remarkably low, the highest being about 12 per cent. for boys of 10½ years. There was no age level at which the interest in collecting and hoarding suddenly increased or decreased. Thus, one investigator found hardly more than 10 per cent. making collections, the other about 90 per cent. What is the explanation of this astonishing discrepancy? The answer seems to be that environmental conditions have changed in the intervening thirty years. Present day conditions offer opportunities to use leisure that are more attractive to the young, such as theatres, moving pictures, wireless, dancing, etc. If an investigation were made to-day cross-word puzzles would shew that a high percentage of children were puzzlers. Conclusions based upon a study of the interest in cross-word puzzles would be applicable only to the time at which the study was made. The parallel with respect to collecting and hoarding activities is obvious. We may reasonably conclude that the collecting instinct is entirely an environmental affair, and not a natural endowment.

Similar remarks apply to any other of the instincts usually named in psychological lists. Thus the fact of war has often been regarded as pointing to an instinct of pugnacity in human beings. And, for this reason, war has even been described as a biological necessity. But a recent school of ethnologists of which Dr Perry and Professor Elliot Smith are the protagonists have brought forward evidence to shew that man was not driven into war by an instinct of pugnacity, but by the growth of organization amongst peoples, with the consequent desire to enslave their neighbours. War, in fact, is a custom and at the present day it is obviously a means whereby governments secure political ends. Again it has been urged that the pressure of population is the stimulus which releases the pugnacious instinct in primitive and civilized communities. But Professor Carr-Saunders in his valuable book on the *Population Problem* (8) has examined the evidence for this view and definitely rejects it. He thinks that wars may have arisen in this way owing to mistaken views of the population problem. That is to say, a theory and not a fact about population is responsible for war ; and there is nothing in the nature of man or of social organization which makes war inevitable. The attribution of war to an instinct is but another instance of the ignoring of sociality with its customs and conventions as the essential feature of human nature.

The fact of the matter is that if we choose to make human activity a question of instinct we can invent as many instincts as we please. Thus the tendency to betting is so widely spread as to constitute a grave social evil. Also any gamester would agree that it has a decided emotional background. Hence this tendency has the distinguishing marks of the other so-called instincts and there ought to be an aleatory instinct. The gratification of this instinct costs all civilized nations a good deal and is reponsible for much ecomonic activity.

But we may go further than the mere enumeration of such specific activities as the aleatory instinct. For it has been urged, with much justification, that thinking itself possesses all the criteria which are supposed to mark off instinctive actions. (15) We saw at the beginning of this chapter that the transparent obviousness of an act, combined with its satisfyingness, are considered good marks of an instinct. Now human thinking is pursued in the same unquestioning way, for we take it for granted and it undoubtedly satisfies our nature. The axioms of logic are quite as inexplicable and acceptable as any instinctive impulse that has been named. Again, nobody would venture to deny that there is an urge towards thinking, since it is frequently carried on in spite of all difficulties and disappointments, to gain no ulterior end except its own worth-whileness. The pursuit of knowledge for its own sake is said to be the distinguishing mark of a philosopher. A further criterion of an instinct, which has frequently been urged as a convincing proof of its forming an essential part of the endowment of the mind, is the pain or annoyance that ensues on its being thwarted. This too is the mark of all intelligent thinking, since nothing is so annoying or disturbing as thwarted thought. And just as instincts, or some of them, have been identified by the accompanying underlying emotion ; so there is always a background of affective tone accompanying successful thinking, as is proved by the fact that obstructed thinking leads to repeated efforts to overcome the obstacles and ultimately to annoyance. The final criterion by which instincts are characterized are their liability to perversions ; and this character, too, can be discerned in thought, since errors and deliberate lying are perversions of the thinking process, just as cruelty may be one of the perverted manifestations of the sexual appetite. We may reasonably assert that, since the criteria by which instincts have been delimited do not serve to separate them from any other mode of activity, the notion of separate instincts is invalid in psychology.

Having thus shewn that the notion of separate human instincts is based on an erroneous analysis of human activity it remains to enquire into the cause of the error, since this has a direct bearing on the mind-body problem. There are three spectres which have pursued us from the beginning of our enquiry into this problem and unless these are definitely laid nothing but confusion can result. One of these has haunted psychology for so long that most psychologists have come to terms with it, namely the faculty theory. The other two are fairly recent intruders and they must be grappled with ; to wit the structural theory of mental life, and the doctrine of mental energy.

Little need be said about the last of these since the previous chapter has been devoted to the topic. There we saw that to talk of the energy ' belonging to a particular instinct ' or ' derived from some instinct ' was to invent a physiology unknown to physiologists. The energy belongs to an individual and is exhibited when he acts ; but each instinct has no specific source of energy. The energy of an animal is not divided up into parcels each available for some specific instinct ; nor are there different qualitative forms of energy assigned to different instincts. The person has the same energy whether he acts in one way or another, *i.e.* any available energy that he

N

has is available for any act of which he is capable. If a man prefers to lift heavy weights rather than row a boat he calls on exactly the same energy in his muscular system. There are not two stores of energy, one for rowing the other for lifting weights. Similarly when a man acts under the motive of fear, anger, or any other assumed instinctive force he uses the same muscular system and the same energy.

Again the notion of separate independent impulsive forces urging men to act in specific ways, which is the theory underlying the belief in instincts, is due in the main to the existence of separate organs for such activities as sex and hunger. The existence of specific bodily organs leads to the view that there are corresponding psychic organs or forces or impulses, owing to the belief in the point-to-point correspondence between body and mind. But no activities, not even the two we have considered in detail, are confined to the organs which are obviously involved in their execution : since the whole organism is concerned to a greater or lesser degree in every act ; internal muscles, circulation, secretions, etc., etc. And as we have now abundantly seen, the quality of the act depends on the nature of the environment and social system. So that the ' feel ' of the act is different on each occasion and there is no one mental impulse underlying all acts which go by the same name.

But a more subtle theory underlies the doctrine of instincts ; which we must now examine. This is borrowed from biology and consists in the belief that the structure of an organ determines its function. It may be worth while, therefore, to consider what view is taken by modern biologists about the relations of function to structure. Mr G. R. de Beer (16) writes " The internal factors of an animal are possessed equally by the cells in all its parts. So the cells of the head of a worm can by regeneration produce a tail, and the cells of the tail can regenerate a head. But if the cells of the head possess the internal factors which control the production of a tail as well as the internal factors which control the production of a head, how is it that in normal development these cells do produce a head and not a tail ? Child has solved this problem by shewing experimentally that the first thing which has to be settled in a developing egg is the polarity, *i.e.* which part of the egg will give rise to the front and which to the hind end of the future animal. Now the determination of this polarity is the result of the action of factors which are *external* to the fertilized egg. All the way through development the internal factors produce nothing of themselves, but they enable the animal to react in definite ways to the external factors and by this means to give rise to structure after structure in the process of development. Heredity does not account for the individual, but merely for the potentialities some of which are realized in the individual.

The same point of view has been developed by Goodrich, who stresses the distinction which has to be drawn between the process of transmission of the internal factors from parent to offspring, and the process of production in the offspring of characters similar to those which were possessed by the parent. An organism is moulded as the result of the interaction between the conditions or stimuli which make up its environment and the factors of inheritance. No single part is completely acquired, or due to inheritance alone. Characters are due to responses and have to be made anew at each generation ".

Here, then, we see that, even on biological grounds, structure is determined by function. And from the psychological standpoint this is a rule without any exception. For such structure or organization as the mind may be said to possess is entirely dependent on subjective functioning. And function must be carried on with reference to some environment. The fact of the matter is, that the notion that mental functioning is due to a particular structure derives its plausibility from mechanical analogies. An engineer could explain some particular action of a machine, not in terms of the action itself, but by reference to the structure of the valves, pistons, rods, cylinders, etc. Similarly it is thought that the activity of the mind can be explained in the same way. But the analogy is most misleading ; for the only knowledge we have or can have of ' mental structure ' is by observing mental activity in ourselves or others. And the only way in which we can describe such structure is by reference to the activity itself. So that from the psychological standpoint ' structure ' is only an indirect way of describing mental functioning. If we take a sufficiently long view the same is true of biological functions. For in the history of organic life digestion appeared before stomachs or even alimentary canals, locomotion took place in diverse ways before limbs were developed, and so on through the whole gamut of activities. Hence it is obvious that phyletically speaking function must have antedated any specialized structure for carrying it out. In other words the course of evolution must have been directed at every stage ; and the theory of lapsed conscious striving is the only plausible explanation that has ever been suggested. (17)

If we must make use of analogies in explaining conscious processes it is always best to derive them from biological functioning. But if we do so we are inevitably thrown back on consciousness itself. The mistake we are trying to eradicate is due to an incorrect view of the nature of mental dispositions. These are regarded by many psychologists, after the analogy of the brain, as a set of enduring psychical structures. But there are many facts to shew that mental dispositions are primarily functional, not structural. Thus, improvement takes place in mental processes, such as memory, when no practice is taken. If we learn a poem late at night we remember it better the following morning. The same thing happens with an annoying problem which sometimes clears itself up if we sleep on it. These, and a host of similar facts, shew that there must be some sort of subliminal functioning during periods of inactivity. Again, as Dr C. S. Myers (18) has pointed out the tendency to ' perseveration ', or the spontaneous recurrence of mental events, is most noticeable in a state of fatigue. This seems to me only explicable on the assumption that when the higher powers of the mind are working badly, or with difficulty, the spontaneous functioning of the mind gets a chance of displaying itself. Hence, it is evident that mental dispositions are functional, not structural.

The third of our spectres remains, and this is the most

insistent, for as Mr J. C. Field (19) has so well shewn the new psychology of instinct is the old faculty psychology masquerading under a new name. He illustrates his remarks by the so-called herd-instinct which is found in cattle ; and sets it against the act of the good Samaritan. What can possibly be the meaning, he asks, of saying that both act from the same instinct? If it is meant that the Samaritan's act is spontaneous well and good. If it is implied that his act, like the cattle's, is not the result of love and sympathy, or is without foresight of the end it is ridiculous. Why then are acts whose conscious concomitants are utterly different ascribed to the same instinct, and what is the good of doing so ? The blunder of the faculty psychology was to subsume diverse acts under one class name, to ignore their differences, and then to attribute to the class so defined a power or activity to produce the acts. Thus every process of imagining was subsumed under the class 'imagination' and then the imagination became the power producing acts of imagining. In this way a mythical structure was placed behind the function. In a similar fashion instincts have been inserted behind certain activities which have nothing but the name in common, and thus the instincts become, by a veritable miracle, mental forces. Professor J. Dewey (20) in his masterly treatise on *Human Nature and Conduct* has exposed the blunder with regard to instinct. He says : " Fear, it will be said, is a reality, and so is anger, and rivalry, and love of mastery of others, and self-abasement, maternal love, sexual desire, gregariousness and envy, and each has its own appropriate deed as a result. Of course they are realities. So are suction, rusting of metals, thunder and lightning and flying machines. But science and invention did not get on as long as men indulged in the notion of special forces to account for such phenomena. . . . They spoke of nature's abhorrence of a vacuum ; of a force of combustion ; of heaviness and levity as forces. It turned out that these ' forces ' were only the phenomena over again, translated from a specific and concrete form (in which they were at least actual) into a generalized form in which they were verbal."

Having laid our ghosts it remains to enquire as to what is

left of the doctrine of instincts. The question may now be reduced to the simple enquiry whether there are any inborn impulses to mental activity. It is necessary to eliminate all reference to reflex activity; since in the first place reflex action is an abstraction as we saw in an earlier chapter, and secondly the mental significance of reflex activity is negligible. What reason then is there to suppose that there are such entities as inborn mental drives? And if such occur is there any reason to suppose that they determine specific activities? The obvious direction in which to look for a primitive mental drive is in the region of appetites. The two strongest appetites are by universal consent hunger and sex. With regard to the latter we have seen that its drive is a matter entirely of custom or social institution. When the sexual organs are mature all that the *untutored* youth feels is a vague restlessness which, in some cases, he is not able even to localize. Custom and tradition determine for him what specific activities will ensue. Sex is a drive, but it is initially entirely blind as to its own means of satisfaction. Similar conditions apply to hunger. From the time that a child is born the satisfaction of this impulse is assured, but there is no reason whatever to suppose that the child is in any conceivable sense aware of what will satisfy the impulse; that is determined for him. Hunger, like sex, is only ' natural ' in the sense that some sort of satisfaction is imperative, but not in the sense that specific activities are ready made and that there is a drive towards these. As Professor Dewey says " only when a man is starving, is hunger an unqualified natural impulse; as it approaches this limit, it tends to lose, moreover, its psychological distinctness and to become a raven of the entire organism." Similar observations may be applied to any other natural appetite. That is to say, psychologically their distinctiveness is acquired and their specific nature is given to them by custom or habit. And the number of such appetites is strictly limited. The only ones that have any strong claim to be included beyond the above two are the appetite to live with others and to derive satisfaction from their presence, the so-called herd-instinct, and the impulse to communicate our thoughts and emotions to our fellows, *i.e.* the language appetite. Possibly we may add to these the appetite for sleep, since there appears to be a strong craving for this, not satisfied in any other way. So that the ' natural ' drives are about a beggarly half a dozen.

If we leave the appetites and ask whether there are any inborn drives outside their range the answer has already been given in the negative in our treatment. But it is worth while, in order to clinch the argument, to consider another so-called instinctive drive, which is invariably included among the inborn impulses ; the emotion of fear. If this cannot be regarded as, in any intelligible sense, an inborn impulse to activity then it is hard to see how any other emotion can have any claim to be so regarded; for fear is the sthenic emotion *par excellence*. Professor J. B. Watson (6) as the result of a study of children in maternity wards attempted to answer the question as to what stimuli, apart from all training, would call out this emotional response. He found that the only situations which called forth fear reaction, at or shortly after birth, were loud sounds, the sudden removal of all means of support or a slight shake when the child is falling asleep or on the point of waking. He was unable to find any trace of an instinctive fear of the dark or of any sort of animal, even of flapping pigeons which present a formidable appearance when close at hand. If we reflect for a moment we see that, in the first year or so of life fear could have no biological value, since the child is helpless. Mr Bertrand Russell by a close observation of his own children has confirmed all this. He too, found no fear of the dark or animals in the first two years of life. All such fears are suggested by the influence of the home environment or imitated from others. (21) For the child is peculiarly suggestible to the response of fear in its elders and readily imitates them in this respect. So subtle is the suggestion that those who are themselves fearful communicate this feeling to children with whom they associate, by slight indications of which they themselves may be unconscious.

For this reason it is very difficult to say what is original and what is acquired in the case of any particular fear. And though loud noises usually do cause fear at any early age they do not invariably do so. (22) Professor C. W. Valentine, who is responsible for this observation on his own children, calls attention to the fear of the ' uncanny ' which some children experience. And similar observations have been made by Mr Russell who found a fear of certain mechanical toys. One would like to know in these cases what suggested the fear. There is one curious fact, difficult to explain, namely that some children find a delight in repeating experiences which they know will cause them fear. This corresponds to the morbid tendency some adults have to read fearful stories even when they dislike them. But the assumption that these fears are inborn rests on no proved foundation.

However, all the observations have shewn that the number of situations which will arouse fear in unspoilt children is remarkably few ; and that the great majority of adult fears are acquired, being explicable as the result of suggestion or other experiences. But it is to be carefully noted that there is no reason whatever to suppose that all such acquired fears have their root in a single instinctive fear. That there is a single impulse or drive behind all fears is a pure assumption. Fears are qualitatively different and not greater or less variations of a single impulse. As has been well said (20) : " There is no one fear having diverse manifestations ; there are as many qualitatively different fears as there are objects responded to and different consequences sensed and observed. Fear of the dark is different from fear of publicity, fear of the dentist from fear of ghosts, fear of conspicuous success from fear of humiliation, fear of a bat from fear of a bear." It is only the difficulty of breaking away from the faculty psychology which could account for the belief that there is one impulse to fear which shews itself in many manifestations, or which supposes that there is a single fear drive which causes all these and other varieties of fear. The class name which includes them all cannot, as was said above, be converted into a ' force ' causing these fears.

There are however acquired impulses or drives to activity. Despite this there has been a tendency for psychologists to deny that habits have propulsive power, owing to the belief that all strong tendencies to action must be instinctive. Consequently habits are supposed to derive such impulsive force as they have from instincts. But since there are no separate instincts and the number of native appetites is strictly limited the view must be rejected. Everybody agrees that bad habits are impulsive forces and the victim of such habits is prone to offer as an excuse that he cannot help himself. The confirmed gambler or drug taker feels an over-bearing impulse to act as he does. And moralists in all ages, recognizing this, have warned the young not to cultivate bad habits as they will inevitably later take control of the person. So that, as far as bad habits are concerned, the union of habit with desire and impulsive force is acknowledged. What is true of bad habits is true of all of them ; and educators have at all times attempted to inculcate desirable habits in the firm and well grounded belief that these will be forces prompting to action all through life. Moreover it would be passing strange if a feature that is characteristic of one set of habits should be lacking in another. A habit, in fact, is a standing predilection or aversion from some specific actions. (23)

This undoubted impulsive power of habit is largely responsible for the belief in separate instincts. In observing the behaviour of human beings psychologists have been struck by the uniformity of action and the strength of custom. To account for the latter they have attributed its strength to the supposed fact that such customs derive their motive power from the native endowment of the mind. But inborn impulses, as we have abundantly seen, are infinitely plastic and such motive power as they possess is entirely the result of the pressure of the social environment which moulds people to its own form.

That there is anything inevitable in such moulding we have given reason to deny ; and consequently there is no reason to believe in an unchanging human nature. Impulses may be organized into almost any dispositions according to the variety of social milieu. Those who object to change always interpret the structure of society as an expression of certain innate human capacities, such as the instinct of acquisition, gregariousness and so forth. But as Professor J. Dewey has pointed out " If we are to shove a mythological psychology of instinct behind modern economics, we should do better to invent instincts for security, a good time, power and success than to rely upon the acquisitive instinct. We should have to give much weight to a peculiar sporting instinct." We may conclude that so far from instincts having any impulsive power over us they derive such force as they have entirely from the habits we cultivate.

Chapter IX

A GREAT ILLUSION

WE have had frequent occasion, during the course of the previous chapters, to call attention to the dogma that the so-called sensory areas in the brain store up mental images. When a sensory experience occurs a sort of deposit is supposed to be left behind, which ensures that internal stimulation shall arouse an image, just as an external stimulus arouses a sensation.

The thesis that it is proposed to elucidate in this chapter is that this is a mistaken view and that all normal people, and especially psychologists, are under an illusion with respect to their mental imagery. What they think they perceive is very different from what they do actually experience. To make this clear we may divide illusions into two classes; those in which the false perception can be corrected by more careful observation, and those in which it is persistent and resists correction. The Müller-Lyer figure, in which two parallel lines appear to meet when they are crossed by other lines, is an example of an illusion which no effort of will can eliminate, even for those persons who are perfectly well aware of the nature of the error and make an effort to counteract it. There is nothing, therefore, paradoxical in the view that an illusion can be universal and persistent, and the apparent certainty of introspective evidence as to what we perceive can be disregarded.

A curious phenomenon, which has never been investigated as far as I know, is that many illusions arise from the fact that the data of one particular sense yield a feeling of an experience from another sense. Thus, several optical illusions are errors of muscular sensibility. The most common and striking of these is the illusion familiar at railway stations ;

when, seated in a motionless train, an adjacent moving train gives us a strong feeling of being moved in the opposite direction ; which feeling, I myself, find it impossible to get rid of by any direct effort of will. Bearing in mind these three characteristics, namely, that an illusion may be universal, that the data from one region of experience are often mistaken for those of another, and that the conviction of complete certainty which the experience carries with it may be erroneous, we are in a position to understand the nature of mental images.

In opposition to the view here maintained there has long persisted a belief that mental images are copies or residua of past sensations. Although a considerable amount of thought has been devoted to the problem of the nature of sensation, few psychologists have faced the question of the nature of mental images. The reason undoubtedly is that images are assumed to be faint copies of sensations, and therefore the ontology of the latter is supposed to carry that of images with them. Now undoubtedly images do occur after we have had the corresponding sensations. But to assume, therefore, that they are copies of impressions is about as reasonable as the view that, because the coolness of night always occurs after the day has gone, the feeling of coolness must be a residuum or copy of the noonday heat.

Even such a careful analytic psychologist as Professor G. F. Stout cannot rid himself of the view that sensations and images are essentially of the same nature. He devotes a long section in his *Manual* (1) to what he calls the characteristic differences of impressions and images ; thereby suggesting that in their essence they are the same. There would be no sense in considering differences between two things which were in totally different categories, such as, let us say, the differences between emotions and images. Professor Stout is not very happy about the matter and tries to make the best of both worlds. For, after considering the difference in intensity between an impression and an image, he concludes that " at bottom the distinction between an image and percept as respectively faint and vivid states, is based on a difference of kind. The percept has an aggressiveness which does not belong to the image. It strikes the mind with varying degrees of force or liveliness according to the varying intensity of the stimulus." This seems to mean that whilst images and impressions are of the same essential nature they are presented to us in a different manner. Again, when he deals with the relative distinctness of the two he says, " the indistinctness of mental imagery is to a large extent of a quite peculiar character. It is different in *kind* from the indistinctness of percepts. . . . An image is sketchy and schematic, because it contains only an extract from the content of sense-perception." Here, again, the substance of the two is supposed to be the same, but the image contains less of it, only an extract. Now I wish to maintain that the difference is not a mere difference in presentation, or sketchiness of the same material, but a total difference in nature. The difference between the two lies in the fact that they are totally different.

The first really scientific study of mental imagery was made by Galton (2) who framed a questionnaire which he submitted to large numbers of people asking them to describe their mental imagery. Unfortunately he started with the tacit assumption that images were faint copies of sensations. Thus, for example, he asked his subjects to describe carefully " the picture that rises before your mind's eye," when thinking of such a thing as the morning's breakfast table. He says that the results of his inquiry amazed him. " To my astonishment, I found that the great majority of the men of science to whom I first applied protested that mental imagery was unknown to them, and they looked on me as fanciful and fantastic in supposing that the words ' mental imagery ' really expressed what I believed everybody supposed them to mean. . . . On the other hand, when I spoke to persons whom I met in general society, I found an entirely different disposition to prevail. Many men and yet a larger number of women, and many boys and girls, declared that they habitually saw mental imagery, and that it was perfectly distinct to them and full of colour." What is really amazing in all this is that such a shrewd person as Galton should have accepted the introspective evidence of untrained observers, including boys and girls, whilst rejecting the more trustworthy statements of cautious scientific men. However, Galton's conclusions still hold sway amongst psychologists, and it is widely held that scientific men and abstract thinkers have feeble powers of mental imagery, having lost the faculty owing to disuse. The sequel will shew that all this evidence is mistaken.

It is necessary, in order to get our ideas clear, to draw a sharp line of distinction between mental imagery and the material of hallucinations and dreams. Unfortunately these are all regarded as being of the same nature. Just as images are supposed to be faint sensations, so dreams and hallucinations are assumed to be vivid images. When Joan of Arc heard real voices she was not necessarily endowed with strong auditory imagery but was under the influence of hallucinations. If such hallucinations are confused with normal images then it would seem that everybody who experiences auditory images must be suffering every day from a mild form of hallucination. I hold that, whenever a hallucination occurs, the corresponding sense organ must, in some way, be stimulated, giving rise to a real sensation. The investigations of ' eidetic imagery ' by Professor E. R. Jaensch (3) have brought to light a new source of hallucinations. He is careful to point out that such ' images ' are actually *seen* in space and are thus distinguished from true memory images. The conditions under which these investigations take place constitute a powerful source of suggestion to immature people, which brings about a state of mind favourable to hallucination. It is thought by Jaensch that eidetic images constitute a link between memory images and sensations. But such hallucinations are, as the sequel will shew, of a totally different nature from images, and it is erroneous to apply the name of images to them. If they really do occur, as stated, they might be called day-dreams in the true sense of the word dreaming.

Hallucinations, like sensations, but unlike images, appear abruptly, or as Professor Stout would say they " strike the mind." They are true sensations, and the only difference between them and other sensations is that no object happens to be present ; that is all. But the sense organs are present and are active. Should the sense organ be absent the stimulation of the sensory nerve is adequate to produce the hallucination. Thus a person who has lost his hand may feel it again if the brachial nerve is electrically stimulated, and he will feel it occasionally when it is stimulated by any form of irritation of the nerve stump. A similar form of stimulation of the sensory organs or sensory nerves is adequate to account for all forms of dreaming. Those who hold the contrary view and think that dreams are constituted of mental images must live in a curious world in the day-time, in which half is dream and half reality. In fact they must always be day-dreaming.

The preposterous error of the assumption that mental imagery is composed of the same stuff as sensations is evident from the following considerations. I cannot see a rose as red at the same time that it appears white, but there is nothing whatever inconsistent in seeing it white whilst at the same time I imagine that it is red. If I look at a white rose, and at the same time imagine it red, the rose still remains white for me. Whereas if an image were a faint copy or an extract of a sensation the rose ought to appear pink. If it does not appear pink then it cannot be the case that, when I imagine it red, I am ' seeing ' anything with my mind's eye. In fact it is impossible for me to understand what is meant by ' seeing ' when I do not use my eyes, or ' hearing ' without ears, and so forth. All this highly metaphorical language about seeing with the mind's eye is most misleading. And only a naïve psychological theory could accept it as a literal expression of what actually occurs. A thing to be ' seen ' must be in space-time but it is hard to believe that images exist spatially. No doubt they appear to be spatially located, but that is part of the great illusion. The confusion between the metaphorical and the real, combined with a strong belief that mental images must have the same physiological basis as sensations in the central nervous system, is responsible for the wide-spread confusion between images, hallucinations and dreams.

Our knowledge of the physiological (as opposed to the anatomical) basis of sensation is not very profound; being limited to the fact that the precursor of a sensation is some organic change in a sense organ, together with some vague knowledge that the different modalities of the same category of sensation are somehow dependent on differences in the terminal part of the sensory apparatus. Our knowledge of the organic basis of imagery is absolutely nil, being confined to guesses as to what ought to be happening in the nervous system. It is absurd, therefore, to found a theory of images on a physiological basis, or to suppose that since they have the same organic basis they must be of the same substance as sensations.

It is, as Professor G. Dawes Hicks (4) has very pertinently observed, in the best study of the nature of images that I am familiar with, " mere mythology to talk of a ' copy ', which a presentation has sloughed off, persisting in some sub-conscious region of the mind, there awaiting in disconsolate exile, until association announces resurrection and recall." John Stuart Mill went so far as to affirm that the difference between a sensation and an image was ultimate; and, but for the fact that there is a temporal relation between them, this view seems to me quite sound.

This supposition, that the occurrence of a mental image is due to some change in the nervous system, might account for the appearance of the image but would give no explanation whatever of its nature. For, as we have said, the nature of mental images is *toto coelo* different from sensations. When we talk of sensations being ' revived ' as mental images the apparently innocent metaphor presupposes our adherence to an idealistic system of metaphysics. It assumes, that is to say, that sensations are purely mental; parts of the mind. To Berkeley (5) it " seemed evident that the various sensations or ideas imprinted on the sense cannot exist otherwise than *in* a mind perceiving them," and the whole choir of heaven and the furniture of earth were, for him, entirely mental. It was open, therefore, to him to assume that sensations could be revived, since what affected a certain medium could leave impressions or traces in that medium. But for anybody who is not an idealist philosopher the whole position is untenable. If sensations never were, from the outset, parts of the mind how is it possible to talk of their mental revival? An impression can leave a trace where it is made and not elsewhere. Characters written on a sheet of parchment may be read centuries later on the parchment, but not on the moon or the stars. Now sensations are not psychologically parts of the mind but are the means by which the mind apprehends objects. In the absence, therefore, of the objects sensations cannot be reproduced mentally nor copies of them, however faint; for this would suppose that the impressions were mental to begin with. We might as well suppose that since images can be seen in a looking-glass, therefore, the looking-glass is able to retain copies when the objects are removed.

On the other hand, in apprehending a sensation there must always be the act of apprehension itself which, being a purely subjective or mental phenomenon, can obviously leave traces of itself in the mind. Where an impression has been made there it can be deciphered; not elsewhere. The act of apprehending can, therefore, leave a mental trace of itself; and in fact this is what it does. I am, therefore, in complete agreement with Professor Dawes Hicks, who has reached the same conclusions as myself by a very different method of approach, when he says: "The contents of our own cognitive acts, the awareness which we live through, these are the mind's own property, or rather go to constitute its very being, and these we are forced to recognize it has the power of retaining in some form and reviving." The sole objection that can be taken to this last remark is the apparent restriction to cognitive acts. For there is even stronger reason to suppose that our affective and conative acts are likewise capable of retention and revival. The act of awareness or apprehending is not simple but a complex mental act in which factors of feeling and conation are integral parts. The cognitive factor is distinguishable, no doubt, by analysis, but is never found in isolation; and the sequel will shew that our emotional states play a prominent part in what appears to be merely cognitive revival.

o

It is desirable, on this ground, to attempt a brief analysis of the process of perception; since whatever the nature of a mental image it must have, as its antecedent, some act of perception. The analysis of perception given by Dr James Drever (6) will help us here. According to his account every act of perception involves not only a sensational element but also an impulse and an interest. As both the interest and the impulse are subjective states they cannot be made the object of direct cognition. The most careful introspection of the objective side of experience, such as might be undertaken for purposes of psychological observation, will reveal nothing but sensational or objective elements in a perceptive act. Nevertheless, there cannot be the slightest doubt that we experience directly both the impulse and the interest, *i.e.* both affective and conative states; we live through them. They are the very tissue of our living experience, without which the world would have no meaning for us. For meaning, in its psychological sense, as opposed to the logical, belongs to the subjective side of experience. And although Dr Drever would probably maintain firmly that we do perceive images, his contention that the primary tissue of experience is composed of meanings rather than of impressions, and that meaning is affective, is quite sound. I would merely add that meaning is both affective and conative. In order that an object should have any meaning for us there must be a reference to something that is in us. But I go further and insist that this something, call it interest or feeling or worthwhileness, or what you will, though by its very nature it cannot be cognized is always *felt*, and can therefore be revived as it is felt. In brief a perceptual experience leaves not only a cognitive, but an affective-conative trace which determines future experience; and this is the only meaning I can assign to its leaving a residuum or copy of itself in the mind.

The events which improve a tennis player's game are the changes made on himself, his muscles, senses and so on; not the impressions which he makes on the ball or the court. This is so obvious as to be childishly trivial. Yet, when we are dealing with mental images, this truism is overlooked or denied. The tennis player, with his muscular and sensory adjustments, corresponds to the act of awareness or apprehension; whilst the court and the balls and all the rest of it may be likened to what is apprehended. What the tennis player permanently carried about with him, after playing, is a more finely adjusted organism. To suppose that sensations in a faint form must be permanent, in order to enable us to remember what has occurred, is equivalent to the supposition that the tennis player must always carry about with him his old balls and racquets in order to improve his play.

Leaving illustrations on one side, what it all comes to is this. When we experience a sensation, or an impression strikes the mind, there are two things to be considered; there is the act of sensing and there is what we sense. The latter is purely objective and non-mental; it is, in short, what confronts us when we are aware of an object. The stuff of which it is composed, is the material, whatever its nature, of which the external world is composed. On the other hand the act of awareness or experiencing is mental, is part of the life history of the person. The stuff of which this is made is experience. Now, in the light of what we have said, it is patent that the only thing which the mind can retain, as the result of its experience, is experience itself, for this is part of the mind. The mind is affected by its experiences and these determine future experience; but we obviously cannot retain what we never had. It is clear that there must be a fundamental qualitative difference between a sensation and an image. In fact it is inadequate to describe it as a qualitative distinction, since there is a difference of category; each belonging to a different realm of reality. A moment's introspection will suffice to convince anybody, not obsessed by any preconceived theory, that the nature of images is totally different from that of perceptions. It needs but to open one's eyes and survey the universe, whilst reflecting on one's images, to see that they are worlds asunder. And what a curious world it would be otherwise, in which objects were located in space-time and copies of them of a fainter kind were jostling them all the while. No doubt we all speak of seeing things with the mind's eye. But this highly metaphorical expression, rightly regarded, so far from deceiving us, ought to keep us to the straight path. Since what is capable of being seen with the mind's eye must be composed of totally different stuff from that which may be seen with the real eye ; mental stuff in fact.

Having assured ourselves that mental images have a different sort of reality from sensations, we must now attempt more closely to investigate the nature of such imagery. We have to fill out the details of what has been, so far, merely sketched. What is revived in imagination are not the primary presentations, but the subjective aspects of our acts of perception ; for the objects to which such acts refer can only be revived by a new presentation similar to the first. Now, there is nothing strange in reviving and becoming aware of a state which originally was purely subjective. There is a process, well known to psychologists, in which our own subjective states are perceived in external objects. This is known as empathy, or feeling ourselves into external objects or events. When we talk of the ' raging sea ' or the ' happy fields ' we actually seem to recognize our own feelings in the external world. Empathy takes place quite unconsciously and is not, as might at first be supposed, a conscious translation of our feelings outwards. Since, then, affective and conative states, which must have originated in ourselves, are normally perceived in the external world there is nothing strange in supposing that our cognitive states may also be, apparently, perceived objectively. This is what I believe to take place when we are said to recall an image. What we revive are our subjective states, and these, having formed an integral part of our original perceptions, lead us to believe that we are having the same objective appearance over again. We revive a part of the original experience and this gives us the conviction that the whole state has been revived, including its objective components. All our mental images, in fact, are illusions. Now the only difficulty in this theory is to explain why so many people are convinced that they do actually revive their sensations, and why it is hard to persuade them that, when they think they perceive an image, they are really only experiencing a revival of subjective states of awareness and feeling.

This difficulty may be resolved by considering the fallibility of the evidence of the senses. When Galton began his enquiry into mental imagery, those who were used to evaluating evidence assured him that he was fanciful in supposing that the kind of images he was talking about had any reality. Whereas people in general society, and especially women and boys and girls, gave him detailed accounts of their images. " The more I pressed and cross-questioned them, professing myself to be incredulous, the more obvious was the truth of their first assertions. They described their imagery in minute detail, and they spoke in a tone of surprise at my apparent hesitation in accepting what they said. I felt that I myself should have spoken exactly as they did if I had been describing a scene that lay before my eyes, in broad daylight, to a blind man who persisted in doubting the reality of vision." These people, and especially the boys and girls, could not doubt the evidence of their images. But we have long since been taught to challenge the evidence of our senses. Why should the evidence of our mental imagery fare any better ?

The value of untrained introspective evidence regarding our mental contents is well-nigh worthless. Yet, with respect to other people's mental imagery, it is the only evidence we can get. There is, and can obviously be, only one way of getting into touch with a mental image, that is by having it. Now all our feelings, our attitudes, our moods and so on are capable of recurring, and the view here maintained is that the revival of these is sufficient to make us believe that what we experience when we have a mental image, is a copy of the primary presentation itself. When the same feeling or mood recurs a person naturally imagines that the surrounding circumstances are likewise the same. In pathological cases strong feelings or emotional states may even produce hallucinations. There are two sorts of hallucinations known to pathologists ; the lilliputian which consists of a world of mannikins, and brobdingnagian where the imagined sensations are of enormous size. Now Dr E. Miller (7) has shewn that these varieties are associated with different affective states. The smaller variety appears to the patient during bright hours when he is in a pleasant state of mind. Whereas when the patient complains of terror his hallucinations are of the gigantic form. If, therefore, the form of imagined sensations can be determined by affective states there is nothing surprising in the assumption that true memory images can so be determined.

We have direct verification of the theory we are maintaining in an illusion which is believed by some people to be almost universal. The phenomenon is known by the name of the illusion of false recognition, or *déjà vu*, and consists essentially in the fact that the person seems to recognize or experience for the second time an assemblage of circumstances which, in reality, are quite novel to him. It was first described, under the name of the sentiment of pre-existence by Dr A. L. Wigan(8) in 1844 in a book called the *Duality of the Mind*. In *David Copperfield*, Dickens wrote of the same experience, as follows : " We have all experience of a feeling that comes over us occasionally, of what we are saying and doing having been said and done before, in a remote time, of our having been surrounded, dim ages ago, by the same faces, objects and circumstances." Wigan referred to the sudden conviction that the scene at which we are assisting, though not previously experienced, has been lived through before, with the same persons in the same attitudes, expressing the same sentiments in the same words. The postures, the expression of countenance, the gestures, the tone of voice all seem remembered though they are being observed for the first time. He gives an instructive example from his own experience, which incidentally illustrates an interesting phase in national psychology. Apparently in those days sentiments were unrestrained and the death of a Royal personage let loose a flood of emotions. When Princess Charlotte died " one mighty all-absorbing grief possessed the whole nation till the whole people became infected with an amiable insanity. No one under thirty-five or forty years of age can form a conception of the universal paroxysm of grief which then superseded every other feeling."

Wigan himself was present at the funeral at Windsor " in a state of hysterical irritability " due to lack of food and rest, and standing about for several hours. The surroundings, the funeral anthem and " the paroxysm of violent grief on the part of the bereaved husband " further aggravated his emotional condition. " In an instant I felt not merely an *impression*, but a *conviction*, that I had seen the whole scene before on some former occasion and had even heard the very words addressed to myself by my neighbour."

Kraepelin has also described his own case. He observed the phenomenon, especially, when he found himself amongst persons who bored him. He would then turn his attention from his surroundings to his own thoughts, when his immediate environment appeared to him to recede and to be felt as if in a dream, and suddenly he was aware of the illusion of false recognition. This was accompanied by a persistent feeling of malaise.

The illusion was carefully investigated by Dr E. Bernard-Leroy (9), who examined all the reported cases and collected a large number of his own. He pointed out that it is not a single object which is falsely recognized, but a complete situation in which all the details appear familiar, and that the situation always appears to have been *lived through*. As one observer, Lalande, put it " If it is a question of a landscape one recognizes not only the chief features but every leaf, every tree, every cloud, every ray of light ; *and usually one feels oneself in the same state and has the same sentiments* as the illusory day of the first perception." (italics mine.) Another characteristic feature is that the experience itself lasts for a very short time, not more than two minutes ; but the person himself is often under the impression that it persists much longer. The feature noted by Dickens, that the situation seems very remote and that everything appears covered with a veil, giving it a dim far-off appearance, is not very common though it does occur.

Every day, by the normal working of our memories, we experience events which have happened before. But such ordinary recollections lack the special emotional tang of the experiences we are describing ; and it is this special character which must be accounted for in any attempt to explain the illusion. What strikes the person is not merely the recognition, but the sentiments, or the emotions induced by the novel situation, which he seems to have felt before. As usually happens with purely psychological phenomena attempts have been repeatedly made to explain the illusion on physiological lines. Thus Wigan supposed that the two cerebral hemispheres worked independently ; one of them might be temporarily asleep when a situation first arose, and then woke up. The first impression, consequently, actually preceded the whole experience ; and this explained the illusion. This ingenious but fantastic physiological explanation, of a cerebral lag of one hemisphere in taking in impressions, has been followed by others no less absurd, but all relying on some supposed peculiarity of the nervous system. This is typical of much physiological psychology. One remark is worth making at this point, namely the implied assumption that our mental life must somehow be mirrored in our organisms ; and as there are two hemispheres there must be two trains of thought. Such an assumed point-to-point correspondence of physical and mental events has no warrant in anything that we know. Here we are furnished with another example of the persistent attempts to insert spurious nervous processes behind patent psychological events. For, it will be noticed, that all the facts are purely psychological, founded on direct experience alone, whereas the theories are physiological and mere guess-work. Mr J. W. Dunne, in his *Experiment with Time* (15), gives an ingenious explanation which has the merit of being psychological. He has a theory that dreams not only recall the past, but can anticipate the future. He believes that when the illusion occurs the experience has really happened before, namely in an anticipatory dream, which has been forgotten in the interval.

As was mentioned previously the illusion is most likely to occur when a person is jaded or fatigued or overwrought or bored ; and, although these conditions are not essential, they predispose a man towards the illusion. Now all these con-

ditions are seed-plots for the arousal of emotional states or
attitudes, or affective moods of various kinds. Here, it seems
to me, we have the psychological explanation of the illusion.
For, when a particular state of affairs is accompanied by a
specific emotion or mood, it is perfectly easy to see that the
subsequent arousal of the emotional condition will have a
tendency to reinstate the original state of affairs. But when
the mood is vague and ill-defined, a mere unanalysable state
of feeling, the attempt at reproduction is likely to be unsuccessful. All that will occur is that we have a vague feeling
that something has happened, we cannot say what. Now
suppose a perfectly new situation to give rise to the same
mood as a previous situation. The person will then have a
feeling that a prior state of affairs has been reinstated. The
logic of the situation (though it must be remembered that
there is nothing reasonable about it, and nothing corresponding
to a judgment of similarity) is that similar feelings tend to
make us believe that the situations are similar. Since we
have the same mood or other emotional state over again we
feel that the situation must be the same. Hence the illusion ;
which is grounded entirely on our affective states of mind and
can have no other origin.

Owing to an intellectual bias in psychology, the importance
of moods, emotions, and obscure organic feelings in determining the train of ideas has not been sufficiently emphasized.
The important part played by contiguity, similarity and so
forth in directing the stream of thought has been often
described. Yet there is no doubt that ideas, which have never
been associated in any of these ways, may recall each other, if
they are connected by a common bond of feeling. When we
are in a joyful mood we can entertain none but rosy ideas,
whereas in a state of grief they stubbornly refuse to present
themselves. Our friends may do their best to bring them
forward but they obstinately refuse to get a lodgment in our
minds. In speaking a foreign language, if we know more
than one, when a word fails us we are apt to supply its
place by an equivalent in some other tongue, not our own.
The reason for this is that, for the time being, we are in the

feeling attitude where only foreign expressions are suggested. G. H. Lewes (10), who commented on this, applied the same explanation to the phenomenon of *déjà vu*, and I have no doubt that he was right. He quotes his own experience, in a foreign land for the first time, when he turned a corner and saw a scene which he could not possibly have seen before. Yet it aroused the vivid conviction that it was already familiar to him. He accounted for it by the fact that the thrill of emotion, which diffused itself over the field of consciousness, obliterated the landmarks whereby new and old would be normally distinguished.

The phenomenon of false recognition is thus due to the fact that certain vague similarities between a present and past situation arouse similar emotional attitudes or moods. The presence of the mood then stimulates a feeling of false recognition. This accounts for the distinguishing characteristic of the illusion, namely that the situation appears, not only familiar, but always to have been lived through. For the essential feature of an affective state is that it is subjective ; something which belongs to the core of the personality. The present impression has a savour or relish of a past one, and this affective similarity gives us a feeling of familiarity which we locate vaguely in the past without being able to assign to it any specific date. One of the early investigators of the phenomenon, E. Boirac, had given a similar explanation and put the matter very clearly. He said : " On peut admettre que toute sensation, toute representation spéciale, surtout quand l'esprit n'est pas encore habitué, est accompagné d'un sentiment propre, d'une saveur (en anglais—*relish*), et ce qu'on pourrait nommer aussi un timbre, une masse affective. Dans le cas qui nous occupe, un object nouveau excite peut-être dans l'esprit, le même sentiment indéfini, innommé, qu'un objet ancien qui ne lui ressemble pas nécessairement et qui est depuis longtemps oublié : d'ou la reconnaissance d'une disposition mentale déjà connue en effet, et l'effort impuissant pour resusciter la perception primitive dont elle faisait partie." (11)

Unexpected experimental confirmation of the explanation we have given has been provided by some experiments on school children, the purpose of which was to discover what advantage moving film pictures had over lantern slides in teaching geography. Both slides and films were shewn representing tea-growing, rubber cultivation, etc., the slides corresponding with parts of the films, both having been taken at the same time. A week after the exhibition each pupil wrote an essay on what he had observed ; and subsequently the same procedure was repeated, with the sole difference that those classes which had the slides now had the films and *vice versa*, thus providing control experiments. It was found that the facts shewn by the optical lantern were more accurately described than those presented by the films. But the interesting result, from our point of view, was that " the control experiments established the fact that often the same children had noticed movements in both films and slides, which goes far to prove that not only the movements in the films *but the mental attitude of the child comes into play* " (italics mine) (12). This independent testimony is valuable as shewing that, in reproduction, the contents of our mental acts play the predominant part. We do not recall passively what is objectively given but the revival is determined by our subjective attitude during presentation. In this particular case the attitude was mainly a conative one. So that both feeling and conation are important factors in recall. As was previously stated, what we retain and revive are the original states of awareness that we have lived through, not the objective things which are presented to us.

A consideration of the psychology of artistic expression confirms the thesis we are maintaining. It was at one time thought that certain subjects or subject matter were artistic, and others not. But Whistler and the early impressionists gave the death blow to this crude belief. An artistic creation is never a faithful copy of the original, and there is no subject which is too trivial or lacking in beauty for the artist. For the artistic product is only partially controlled by the subject matter, depending mainly for its expression on the artist's store of thought and feeling. A faithful copy of what is presented is never the artist's ideal. Professor S. Alexander (13) has an attractive theory of artistic creation which emphasizes this aspect of the process, though he would probably repudiate the theory we are putting forward. He maintains correctly that " the emotion which a work of art exists to communicate is the aesthetic emotion from which the artist created " and *not* " the emotion appropriate to the subject matter which was the artist's stimulus to production." Hence, he insists, that it is vital to distinguish the images excited by the subject-matter from the images of the artistic product itself. Any portrait painted by a master is a complete justification of this standpoint, since nobody could suppose that those who get their portraits painted by eminent artists are more beautiful than those who are painted by minor people. Velasquez' Spanish Admiral was no doubt a repulsive person physically, but that did not prevent the artist from creating a great portrait of him. This may be expressed tritely by saying that the artist always puts part of himself into what he creates. Professor Alexander goes beyond this, and insists that the artist only finds himself when he expresses himself in his peculiar mode of art. He only knows definitely what his own emotions are when he has elaborated them into some artistic product.

This putting of ourselves into what we imagine constitutes, to my mind, the essential core of mental imagery. The resemblance between a mental image and that of which it is incorrectly said to be a ' copy ' consists primarily in the fact that the emotional and conative factors in the image are those which constituted part of the original experience. I do not ' see a thing with my mind's eye ' though I imagine that I do so. But I do experience an emotional attitude over again, which was once part of my experience. This makes the image resemble its original. Whenever I do actually ' see ' something which is not there to see, my physical eyes, the only ones I possess, take part in the process and then I suffer from a hallucination. Mental images are all illusions of a peculiar kind. In a normal illusion I mistake one physical object for another ; whereas when I have a mental image I mistake an affective disposition for a physical object. That is all; and the rest is simply due to faulty introspection. When, therefore, we read remarkable accounts of the rich and varied imagery which some people claim to possess we may be sure that they are endowed with a high degree of affectivity. If it is the case, as is frequently said, that women possess better mental imagery than the majority of men, and that children too are endowed with vivid imagery, we have good evidence that women and children are normally more under the influence of emotion than men.

The theory here maintained, namely that images have no 'body' unless the sense organs are stimulated may be further proved, if necessary, from the evidence of those who live, as we say, in an imaginary world and are capable of describing their experiences correctly. Thus, Anthony Trollope (14) tells us in his *Autobiography* that, as other boys refused to play with him, from the age of twelve he contracted the habit of "always going about with some castle in the air firmly built within my mind. For weeks, for months, from year to year I could carry on the same tale. . . . I learned in this way to maintain an interest in a fictitious story, to dwell on a work created by my own imagination, and to live in a world altogether outside the world of my own material life. In after years I have done the same." His novels were all created in this imaginary world and everyone will agree that his characters are sharply individualized and his descriptions vivid. An unwary psychologist reading this account, and his novels, would assume that he must have had sharp visual pictures in his mind. Yet he himself apparently only saw his characters clearly when Millais drew them for him. This is what he says : " I have carried on some of those characters from book to book and have had my own early ideas impressed indelibly on my memory by the excellence of his delineations." How could this happen if he had already had these pictures in his mind ? The fact that Millais' illustrations struck him as excellent can only mean that his affective disposition waited for good drawings before taking on a body.

What has now been demonstrated in a variety of ways may be briefly summarized. We have seen that it is a characteristic of many illusions that they are universal and unconscious. The evidence of our senses, though in these cases it is palpably false when measured by an objective standard, is too powerful to be corrected by any effort of will. The conviction that we are living through a particular specific experience, though it is demonstrably untrue, cannot be eliminated by any conscious process. An equally striking feature of some illusions lies in the fact that the evidence of one sense is felt or experienced as though it belonged to some other sense, as for example in the illusion of the moving train. And here, too, no effort of will is capable of correcting the feeling.

In both these respects images behave like illusions. Those who have them are perfectly convinced that they are what they seem, and any attempt to shake this belief is foredoomed to failure. Unfortunately it is not possible to provide any objective demonstration of the falsity of their conviction, as it is, for instance, in the example of the Müller-Lyer illusion. Nevertheless, with whatsoever assurance they hold the belief that they see, hear, feel or otherwise experience objects ' in the mind ' anybody who has considered the evidence I have provided must refuse to give credence to their introspective certainty. Nobody who has experienced the moving train illusion can doubt for a moment that the conviction that a particular sense is being stimulated is false, even if it is impossible to shake off the illusion. One mode of experience can so successfully simulate a totally different one that only indirect evidence can inform us of what is really happening. This may help to explain why it is impossible to persuade those who claim to have real objective imagery that they are the victims of an illusion. For, in their case, the illusion is a more subtle one, since they are misinterpreting affective and conative experiences for cognitive impressions. The evidence we have brought forward shews that it is quite common to do this, and yet remain under the delusion that we are doing something else. And further, since our affective states are purely subjective, any attempt to find a physiological basis for mental imagery is foredoomed to failure. When our body dies all possibility of sensations dies with it, but there is no reason whatever to suppose that a like fate overtakes our images or ideas, since these are subjective phenomena in no way dependent on the organism. To this we shall return in the last chapter.

We may conclude that mental images have a different sort of reality from the sensations that we hourly experience ; which is the thesis we set out to justify. The substance of images, the material of which they are composed is not the residua of sensational experience ; but the feelings, moods and conative attitudes which were the accompaniments of the original sensations. And any statement to the contrary, no matter how firmly attested, or held with whatsoever strong introspective conviction, is evidence of a great illusion.

CHAPTER X

EDUCATIONAL PSYCHOLOGY

THE nature of mental activity is obviously a fundamental topic in considering the mind-body problem. Now this subject has been widely investigated by educational psychologists in dealing with the doctrine of mental discipline, or the so-called transfer of the effects of training. To make the point of the discussion clear I will first treat the history of this doctrine, by summarizing what I have said in my *Educational Psychology*. (1)

In the seventh book of Plato's *Republic* the following speech is put into the mouth of Socrates. " Those who have a natural talent for calculation are generally sharp at every other kind of knowledge ; and even the dull, if they have had an arithmetical training, although they may derive no other advantage from it, always become much sharper than they would otherwise have been." Socrates is also reported to have believed that there is an infinite difference between the man who has studied mathematics and the man who has not. Thus he says " We know, of course, that the man who has studied geometry will be wholly and entirely superior to the man who has not, with respect to the better apprehension of all subjects."

This notion of mental discipline persisted throughout the ages ; and Bacon in his essay on *Studies*, doubtless influenced by Plato, propounded it thus : " Nay, there is no stond or impediment in the wit, but may be wrought out by fit studies ; like as diseases of the body may have appropriate exercises. . . . So if a man's wit be wandering, let him study the mathematics ; for in demonstrations, if his wit be called away never so little, he must begin again. If his wit be not apt to distinguish or find differences, let him study the schoolmen ; for they are splitters of hairs."

John Locke put the kernel of the matter very precisely. " I have mentioned mathematics as a way to settle in the mind a habit of reasoning closely and in train ;   not that I think it necessary that all men should be deep mathematicians, but that, having got the way of reasoning, which that study brings the mind to, they might be able to transfer it to other parts of knowledge as they have occasion." In short, the effects of training are of a general nature and not confined to the subject in which the training is received. This is the doctrine of mental discipline, and it obviously raises the whole question of the nature of mental activity. For, if the theory is sound, the received doctrine of specific mental dispositions must be invalid.

In the great controversy in England in the middle of the nineteenth century concerning the claims of natural science, mathematics and modern languages to be included in the school curriculum the warfare raged chiefly round this doctrine of mental discipline or ' transfer of training ' as it came to be most inaptly named. The study of classics was regarded as a species of mental gymnastics, a method of developing the intellectual faculties in general. The Schools Inquiry Commission (2) in 1868 reported that " Nothing appears to develop and discipline the whole man so much as the study which assists the learner to understand the thoughts, to enter into the feelings, to appreciate the moral judgment of others. . . . Nothing contributes to remove narrowness of mind so much as that clear understanding of language which lays open the thoughts of others to ready appreciation. Nor is equal clearness of thought to be obtained in any other way. Clearness of thought is bound up with clearness of language, and the one is impossible without the other." It must be remembered that when the Commissioners spoke of language they meant Latin and Greek. The reason they gave for preferring the classics was the fulness and precision of the accidence which no modern language could rival. And they stated that all schoolmasters were agreed that nothing teaches English grammar so easily or well as Latin grammar, and next to that some other foreign grammar, such as French. One enlightened

P

witness, Earl Fortescue, put the argument in favour of French as a rival to Latin thus : " I believe that the subtler parts of French grammar afford a very good discipline to the mind, and a very fair test of what might be called scholarship in the case of those who have only a limited number of years to bestow on their education." There you have it ; nothing could be clearer. But the protagonists of mathematics and science put forward exactly the same plea for their own studies, asserting that these gave an equally sound mental discipline. It is desirable therefore to examine the theory that the effects of training in one sphere of mental activity can be, as Locke said, transferred to other spheres.

Educational psychologists have made various attempts for nearly forty years to put this conception of mental discipline to the test of experimental investigation. At first sight this seems a rash procedure, since the time involved in bringing any disciplinary influence to bear in the mind must necessarily be a matter of years ; whereas investigations of the kind we are about to consider occupy, at most, only a few weeks. Nevertheless the methods pursued and the results obtained justify us in considering the bearing of this topic on the mind-body problem.

The general method of procedure is to divide a number of persons into two groups or teams of equal ability with reference to some particular capacity. These equivalent groups are selected on the basis of certain specific tests aimed at measuring certain simple capacities. The giving of this set of tests is called taking the first cross section. One of the groups now acts as a control group, whilst the other is trained intensively with reference to the capacity to be investigated. At the end of the period of training a set of tests of exactly the same kind as the first is given, and the ability of the initially equivalent groups is again determined. This second test is called taking the second cross section. It was hoped, in this way, to determine whether or not there was some differential improvement in capacity of the trained group compared with the control group ; whether in other words the effects of the training were specific or generalized. Thus, suppose we started with two groups of equal ability in memorizing verse, and trained one of them to memorize nonsense syllables ; would this make the group as a whole more efficient in memorizing verse than the control group which had received no such training ?

The amount of research devoted to this problem by educational psychologists is overwhelming, but it is by no means easy to evaluate it since the results are so contradictory. It is also necessary to state that most of the work, especially the earlier investigations, was concerned with the ability to perform very simple operations such as the perception of form, simple motor habits, memory, especially of the mechanical kind, and so on. In fact the investigators used the material which they found ready to hand in psychological laboratories, *i.e.* largely of a sensory or motor kind. Amongst the first investigations were those of Professors E. L. Thorndike and R. S. Woodworth. (3) They made a great variety of experiments upon the results of training in estimating areas, lengths, and weights, of certain shape and size, upon the ability to estimate areas, lengths and weights, similar in shape but different in size, different in shape but similar in size, and different in shape and size. Also they estimated the influence of training in various forms of perception upon slightly different forms. The conclusion reached as a result of these careful experiments has been widely accepted and firmly held until to-day, namely, that improvement in any single mental function does not improve the ability in any function closely allied to it. A review of all this earlier work of which there is an enormous volume is given in my *Educational Psychology*. (1)

It has been objected to all these earlier experiments on the topic that the persons experimented on were not sufficiently interested in the artificial laboratory procedure and that, therefore, they had no incentive to do their best. In order to overcome this objection an investigation has more recently been made on the following lines. A certain number of boys of 15 to 18 years of age were engaged from an employment bureau, and divided into two equivalent groups, on the basis of a number of very simple tests in manual dexterity. The tests were devised so as to correspond to the different parts of a very simple operation of a repetitive kind in the chain industry. One of the groups was trained for a fortnight, working six hours a day, in the specific operation, and paid a wage plus a bonus on the amount of improvement effected each day. A bonus was also paid to each group for improvement in the tests. Cross sections were taken by means of the same tests at the end of each week. It turned out that there was no significant difference between the control group and the practised group in the intermediate and final tests. The experimenters concluded that training in manual dexterity of a very mechanical kind is specific rather than general ; which implies that one kind of mechanical skill does not affect others. (4)

This conclusion means that every faculty of the mind is purely specific, and consequently that all training is limited in its results to the material on which the practice is acquired. Such a view is in accord with the theory of mental dispositions as consisting of isolated mental structures ; and more especially with the view which bases skill on the acquirement of certain brain centres. Since such centres are specific, training too must be specific. It is quite true, of course, that a tea taster who has developed his palate so as to be able to detect fine variations in qualities of tea has probably not thereby acquired the palate of a wine bibber. Nor is it likely that a letter sorter who can easily discriminate letters of an ounce or more, by handling, would be able to detect differences of weights where the standard was a pound. As, however, where higher faculties are involved, such a denial of the doctrine of mental discipline appears to be in opposition with the most patent facts of observation, a theory has been devised to account for those cases in which the effects of training are apparently generalized. The theory asserts that generalized training is a delusion, due to insufficient analysis. Thus Professor E. L. Thorndike (5) writes : " One mental function or activity improves others in so far as and because they are in part identical with it, because it contains elements common to them. These identical elements may be in the stuff, the data concerned in the training, or in the [mental] attitude, the method taken with it. The former kind may be called *identities of substance* and the latter, *identities of procedure.*" It is supposed to be owing to these objective or subjective identities that what appears to be a generalized effect of discipline is really only a disguised specific effect, whose specificity is masked by a lack of analysis.

If we consider what the theory implies we see, at once, that to call a particular mental attitude in dealing with a specific situation an identical element in that situation is merely a play upon words. If the attitude adopted by a person in dealing with a new situation is similar to that which he has been trained to adopt in other situations, then his mind has been disciplined and the effects of training have been transferred or generalized. There remains, therefore, to consider only those cases in which the subjective attitude is different but the situation contains identical objective elements.

Fortunately this is a matter which has been submitted to experimental investigation and the results shew that the notion of identical objective elements has no justification. The whole theory, in fact, is based on the supposition that we can consider the behaviour of an animal in physiological terms of stimulus and response. It was demonstrated, in an earlier chapter, that there is no ground for this hypothesis. In some recent experiments on guinea pigs (6) the animals were trained to run down one of two bays in order to secure food. At the end of each bay there was a door containing an illuminated square of opal glass, the size of which could be varied, and the squares were of different sizes in each bay. The animals were trained to choose the bay containing either the smaller or the larger illuminated square and were rewarded, when successful, by being fed. Let us call the door which led to the food the ' positive ' one, the door which was locked the ' negative ' one. The animals rapidly acquired this simple skill. Thus, they were trained to respond to a positive 3-inch square as opposed to a negative 1-inch square. The day after this training was successfuly accomplished the negative 1-inch square was removed and an 8-inch square substituted for it.

Now the identical element in the new situation is the positive 3-inch square. If the theory we are examining is correct, then the animals should have responded to the identical element. But it was found that, in defiance of their practice, they now treated the old positive stimulus as the negative stimulus, and went to the new square, which bore the same sort of relation to the old positive as that bore to the old negative. In brief they responded to the *meaning of the new situation* as a whole, and not to any 'elements' into which the situation may be analysed by an outside observer. By ignoring the positive stimulus, to which they had been trained to respond, they shewed that they understood the new situation, and fully earned the piece of carrot they found behind the door. The experimenter summed up his observations on the animals' behaviour by stating that "it is not possible to account adequately for the animals' behaviour in terms of reactions to isolable elements or sensation units considered in abstraction from each other." An admirable statement; but quite in conflict with any theory about brain centres or specific mental dispositions.

Similar results had been previously obtained by Professor W. Köhler (7) in his well-known study of the mentality of apes; and he concluded, rightly, that the whole attempt to explain behaviour in terms of stimulus and response is artificial. He maintains, and I agree with him, that there are no identical elements, from the psychological point of view, in different situations. What an animal or a person responds to is, as we shewed in an earlier chapter, the meaning or significance of a whole configuration; and the procedure adopted on successive occasions in dealing even with the same situation is never the same. We cannot intelligibly investigate an animal's behaviour unless we assume that it is intelligent If an animal can behave differently in a new situation, ignoring the positive stimulus and reacting only to its relational significance, *i.e.* to the meaning, it is odd to believe that a human being is not capable of doing the same. In the chapter on language we saw that it was erroneous to suppose that a word could be psychologically isolated from its context, and that the artificial attempt to do this destroyed its linguistic value. Similarly we cannot isolate a stimulus from a total situation and assume that there is a response to this alone. Here, once more, physiological conceptions of nerve cells and centres have served to distort psychological facts.

Since the experiments on animals, to which we have referred, shew that transfer of ability does take place ; and since the notion of identical elements in different situations has been shewn to be unsound ; it remains to enquire into the subjective attitude as a possible cause of transfer. Several recent investigations have approached the problem from this angle, with results different from those recorded above. A couple of these may be mentioned.

Mr H. Woodrow (8) dealt with three equivalent groups of college students, one of which was a control group. The initial and final cross sections were obtained by various memory tests of a purely mechanical kind. Two of the groups were given a month's practice in learning verse and nonsense syllables. Whilst, however, one of the groups simply had this mechanical practice all the time, the other group devoted their practice periods partly to discussions on the technique or memorizing, using the rules which psychologists have discovered as most appropriate for memorizing, and applying them. They were encouraged to adopt the technique suggested, which was illustrated by copious examples. It was found that there was no significant difference in the final cross section between those who had the unenlightened drill in memorizing and the control group who had no practice. Whereas, there was a vast difference in favour of the group who had the intelligent practice. It is to be noted that the tests by which the cross sections were taken were of a purely mechanical sort of memory. Hence this investigation makes it evident that intelligent practice, or training enlightened by principles, even in a mechanical ability, is likely to improve that ability in other directions not specifically trained. The experimenter concluded that the great superiority was due " to using the drill material primarily as material with which to conduct practice in proper methods of memorizing and, further, by explaining these methods and calling attention to the ones which should be employed when new kinds of memorizing were undertaken."

Hence if a course of instruction in mathematics (say) produces but little improvement in the ability to reason in other spheres of activity, that tells us very little about the value of mathematics as a means of improving reasoning ability in general. It may simply mean that the course has given practice of a purely mechanical kind. As Professor A. N. Whitehead (9) has well said : " The reason for the failure of mathematics to live up to its reputation is that the fundamental ideas are not explained to the student disentangled from the technical procedure which has been invented to facilitate their exact presentation in particular instances. Accordingly, the unfortunate learner finds himself struggling to acquire a knowledge of a mass of details which are not illuminated by any general conception. Without a doubt, technical facility is a first requisite for valuable mental activity, but it is an error to confine attention to technical processes, excluding consideration of general ideas." A course of mathematics given in an enlightened manner by a teacher who was primarily concerned, not with technical skill and manipulations, but with the principles and ideals aimed at by great mathematicians might produce a general effect on reasoning ability. For what we value that we strive to attain. It is a mistake therefore to consider the educational values of subjects of study *in abstracto*. No subject has a value *per se*, since all depends on the manner of tackling it, whereby a desire is created in the pupil to excel in it. The value of a subject for general education thus depends entirely on the manner in which it is handled, and on the ability of the teacher to make clear to the pupil that the underlying principles are of great and intrinsic worth.

It has become the custom to deride a liberal culture largely because of the unwarranted claim made during the middle of the nineteenth century that the classics alone provided a liberal education. For this reason both the terms ' liberal ' and ' culture ' have gone out of fashion. But if we realize that the educational value of a subject is not some quality inhering in it, but lies in its mode of treatment, we see that almost any subject may be an element in a liberal culture, provided that it is capable of evoking ideals by an insight into principles. By the beginning of the twentieth century educational psychologists had, as we have seen, convinced themselves that training in one mental activity exercised no appreciable influence upon other mental activities, even where these activities seemed to be most immediately akin. The claims of natural science to a place in the curriculum of schools had been universally acknowledged. But it was believed, and is still widely held, that these claims are justified solely on account of the content of science subjects and their great value in promoting practical progress. As the old faculty psychology was by this time dead, it was thought absurd to claim for science any other educational value, such as training the observation, or the powers of inference, in general. The study of chemistry could train a boy to be observant with respect to chemical phenomena, and the study of physics to make inferences about the physical world. The dread of being mistaken for a faculty psychologist prevented any wider claim for these subjects in the sphere of mental activity. But the claim is by no means unjustified.

Much light has been thrown on this whole problem by a recent investigation conducted in a school (10), the importance of which justifies a fairly detailed account. The master, who conducted the investigation, set out to enquire whether by making explicit reference to the methods of science when teaching it, such methods could engender an ideal. To do this he selected one specific feature of scientific method, namely the construction and formulation of precise definitions ; for, in the elaboration of scientific theories, definition is essential. Sixty boys were selected and divided into three groups of twenty, of equal average intelligence, on the basis of intelligence tests combined with the estimates of their capacity by the masters. All the boys were given a set of twenty words in ordinary use to define. The criteria of a good definition, given in the standard works on logic, were taken as the basis for marking this test and securing the first cross section ; such as, that the definition should be by class and difference, should include all that the word means and exclude all else, should not be redundant, and so forth. The boys, of course, did not know on what principle the papers were marked.

One of the groups acted as a control, and the other two groups had a short course on magnetism, which was part of their regular school work. With both of these groups the matter treated in the lessons and the experimental work were precisely the same. After the first lesson the pupils in both groups were asked to define a magnet, and the definition was discussed in the light of what they had learnt about magnetism ; and thence a model definition was reached. One of the groups went no further into the question of definition, but the other group discussed the proper logical form of definition and the various rules indicated above. This was illustrated in a later lesson when the question of the proper definition of ' magnetic induction ' was dealt with and thoroughly treated. The difference, then, between the two trained groups lies in the fact that the one group were trained in the process of defining and a critical analysis of actual definitions, whilst the practice in definition obtained by the other group was merely incidental ; no attention being paid to the process of definition as such.

At this stage a second cross section of all the three groups was taken, by giving them a further set of twenty ordinary words to define, similar to those used in taking the first cross section. Let us call the control group A, the group which had the science lessons but no critical practice in defining B, and the group which had critical practice in analysing definitions C. It was found that the difference in the second cross section between A and B was statistically insignificant, whilst that between A and C was very considerable. In other words the group C had transferred their ability gained in science to dealing with words in ordinary discourse. Although the length of time the investigation lasted was not enough, nor the numbers of pupils sufficiently large to make the inference absolutely certain, we may yet agree with the investigator that when the principles of scientific method are brought to the focus of consciousness science may become a powerful instrument for training the mind to reason aright. We may also infer that practice alone, without conscious rectification, only serves to confirm the person in whatever right or wrong attitudes he may have unconsciously acquired.

It is now time to attempt to evaluate the experimental work which we have considered and to see what conclusions are suggested for the mind-body problem. In the first place it is obvious that all the experimental work is quantitative ; and this is natural, as experiments are devoted to estimating increased facility in certain activities, and the qualitative aspect must be ignored, since it is not measurable. When the attempt is made to measure the improvement in a certain capacity we must rely on the time records, the amount of improvement or the diminution in the number of errors ; all of them quantitative aspects of the capacity examined. Thus if we are trying to discover whether a person's memory has been improved we must find out whether he remembers more with a given number of repetitions, or whether he retains the material for a longer time, or makes less mistakes, and so forth.

But it is clear that a capacity or skill may be trained or improved by organizing our primary abilities in a different manner or by modifying the constituent abilities. In order adequately to describe the effects of training, such qualitative changes are, at least, as important as the quantitative ones. And there are large departments of human activity where quantitative considerations do not apply ; such as in all critical or æsthetic appreciation. Moreover, even where the quantitative aspect is prominent, qualitative considerations may make all the difference. Two persons may solve the same mathematical problem accurately, but the solution of one may be neater or prettier, as we say, than the other. It is the great merit of the *gestalt* school of psychology to have shewn that a situation or a problem is something quite different from the parts into which it may be analysed ; it is a unitary whole. And the solving of a problem, or the coping with a presented situation, rests on insight into the meaning of the configuration considered as a whole. Such insight may produce quantitative effects, but it need not do so ; for it may shew itself, and usually does, in a totally different manner of dealing with the situation.

Most of the earlier experimental work, to which we called attention, was concerned with such simple operations as could be rendered habitual and mechanical by practice. As Professor T. H. Pear (11) has pointed out, when practice has been hardened into a habit the latter, as it were, becomes dissociated from the personality. Such simple habits are almost, but never completely, under the control of the body. This applies to all simple skills, but as I have shewn in *Educational Psychology*, the mind is always the final controller and guider of the process. Still, as the body has taken over most of the vegetative functions, it tends, too, to take over habitual functions, such as speech. And for this reason a person may speak in his sleep. When, therefore, a particular skill is crystallized into a series of habits the possibility of transferring the effects of training is greatly decreased. For the body cannot generalize. Hence the possibility of transfer resulting from the mechanical practice of some simple function is negligible ; and experimental observations as we have abundantly seen bear this out.

But this is only part of the story. Suitable exercise of some mental function may breed not only increased capacity in that direction but a sentiment towards some activity. The person may be stimulated to desire this particular activity, to value it, and to seek to excel in it. If he does so, his whole mental attitude undergoes a change. Should the training be of such a nature as to exhibit the methodological aspects of the study then an ideal may be evoked. It is no longer the facility or activity *per se* which the person desires, but some value, which he can only acquire by means of the practice. The motive for strenuous activity is thus implanted in his mind.

The history of civilization amply shews that the strongest motives to human actions are ideals, which, by breeding a divine discontent, enable a person to overcome the most formidable obstacles. We see, then, that the function of a liberal education, as far as the curriculum is concerned, is not primarily to produce skill in particular subjects but to implant general principles and so engender ideals. If this is done then the whole mental outlook is changed. Any belief to the contrary is founded on an atomic view of the constitution of the mind. Regarded thus, it is of course difficult to imagine how a particular training can influence general ability. But if we consider the nature of an ideal it is quite easy to see how the mind may be steeped and dyed by what it works in. Mr B. Russell tells us that " I can remember a sense almost of intoxication when I first read Newton's deduction of Kepler's Second Law from the law of gravitation." A study which can produce such an effect must surely affect the whole mind, and not merely the ability to reason mathematically ; and Mr Russell, no doubt, owes his reputation in other spheres of activity to the value he attaches to mathematical reasoning.

The attempt to treat the study of mind as purely a natural science has been responsible for many blunders, but hardly for one greater than this we are considering. For though the categories of worth or value are outside the range of scientific treatment there can be no manner of doubt that values are amongst the most powerful of the springs of conduct of human beings. All that psychology can attempt to do here is to try to explain (if it can) how the notion of value or worth arises in the individual. But as to the inner meaning of this concept psychology has nothing to say. It is, in fact, extra-psychological; and yet it affects human volition.

Instincts or other native impulses are sometimes regarded as the sole springs of conduct. But what is patent to the most casual observation is that ideas and ideals have always moved nations and individuals. Here, then, we have the fact, explain it how we will, that a force which is outside the range of natural science is capable of being the most powerful mover of men. Every great department of study is thus capable of influencing the whole personality ; and all real education is thus general and not specific. If then purely non-material, and I may add non-mental forces, are able to produce effects on the mind-body we see that the problem of the relation of the mind to the body has been unduly narrowed. The only way of avoiding the difficulty is to claim that ideals are mental. Now undoubtedly ideals must be known or appreciated before they can function as motives to conduct. But this simply proves they must be presented to some mind. Their existence, however, appears to be entirely independent of the persons to whom they are thus presented. They are, like the Platonic Ideas, not denizens of this world at all; but they are real enough, or how else could they affect conduct and change a man's whole outlook. If education has as its supreme aim the inculcation of ideals then the attempt to formulate it in terms of scientific categories is doomed to failure. We must agree that what has been shewn to be impossible in the realm of nature, namely, to secure a general mental change as the result of specific training, is not only possible but of daily occurrence in the realm of ends.

I cannot do better than quote the late Professor James Ward (12) in this connection : " More life and fuller achieved by much toil and struggle, an ascent to higher levels not movement along the line of least resistance—this is the one increasing purpose that we can so far discern, when we regard the world historically as a realm of ends in place of summarizing it scientifically under a system of concepts. . . . But where in what is, in what we have so far attained, can we discern those eternal values that point upwards and beyond this present world ? Surely in all that we find of the beautiful and the sublime in this earth on which we dwell and the starry heavens above it ; in all that led men long ago to regard nature as a cosmos ; in all that is best and noblest in the annals of human life ; in these very needs themselves that the seen and the temporal fail to meet."

Thus our argument has led us to the following position. Prolonged experiment has demonstrated that when we are dealing with simple skills, or with other activities of a more or less mechanical nature, the training is limited to making us more efficient in these particular matters. Repetitive work in a factory can have no other effect than to make the worker more efficient in repetitive work. It is possible to get some sort of explanation of this result on the basis of bodily mechanisms, but the explanation is only partial and ignores all the difficulties that were referred to in earlier chapters.

Where, however, the work is of such a nature or treated in such a way that it evokes a sentiment or an ideal a different state of affairs emerges. The improvement is no longer confined to the subject we are dealing with but extends to all our other mental activities : we work on a different plane. If the ideals are arrived at by the person himself we speak of inspiration ; and rightly so, since the attempt to explain creative activity on the basis of the analytical-descriptive concepts of psychological science is utterly absurd. Inspiration is derived from a different sphere of reality, the realm of ends. We thus see that the concept of mental activity is unintelligible unless we call in aid the spiritual realm to redress the balance of the psychological world.

CHAPTER XI

MIND MATTER AND PHILOSOPHERS

HAVING elucidated the concept of mental activity we are almost in sight of our goal, namely, the consideration of the relation of body to mind. Yet there remain a few more obstacles to overcome. The problem of the relation of body to mind is usually interpreted to mean the relation of matter to mind. But we have no reason to suppose, at the outset, that these two problems are identical, and the perplexities of the latter problem have obscured the study of the former. We must endeavour to get our ideas clear by separating the two at the beginning, even if we have to unite them at the end. In order to see how the trouble arose it is neceaasry to go back to primitive ideas. The distinction between soul and body was, in primitive thought, a theory about the nature of death. A man was alive and is now dead ; but his body has much the same appearance as before, except that it has lost all power of feeling and motion. The soul was conceived as a sort of subtle body, somewhat in the likeness of dream appearances, but lacking ponderosity. And when it left the body the latter died. Thus Homer conceived the soul as an image in the form of the body, escaping at the moment of death either through the mouth or a wound, and thereafter existing as a shade. The distinction between soul and body was not a distinction between substances one of which was material and the other spiritual ; rather one was an attenuated copy of the other.

The kind of reasoning above exemplified is, according to Sir J. G. Frazer, the method widely adopted by savages. (1) As the savage commonly explains the powers of inanimate nature by supposing that they are produced by living beings working in or behind the phenomena ; so he explains the process of life itself. As a man lives and moves, what is more natural than to suppose that there is a little man inside him who provides the motive power? The man inside the man is the soul. During sleep this inner man goes off on journeys, the evidence of which is to be found in dreams. For, in these, the man does astonishing things which he would not, or could not, do in his waking hours. Death is the result of the permanent absence of the inner man or soul. This mode of explaining the phenomena is not, however, confined to savages or primitive thought. It is, anyhow, more intelligible to conceive of a little man inside doing things than to talk of images or ideas carrying out their own purposes inside the head. Both physiologists and psychologists, who pride themselves on being up to date, talk of images acting in astonishing ways, slipping past the censor and carrying on various other antics. These images, in fact, are conceived as little gnomes or Pucks and can perform the most lively evolutions, all of their own volition.

It is important to bear in mind, that the distinction between the material and the mental is neither primitive nor obvious, as our modern thought is warped by the idea that there are two totally distinct and independent entities which have, somehow, to be reconciled. So far is this from being the natural way of looking at the problem that it was quite late in the history of thought before it was even formulated. Thus Parmenides (2) is reported to have explained all psychological phenomena by the mixture of substances in the body; and drew no distinction between the mental and the corporeal. And some of the Pythagoreans, like some modern scientists, sought the soul in particles that were in motion. This frankly materialistic view, if the name is applicable where the mental was not yet conceived, was also held by Democritus, for whom the soul was a mobile substance pervading the whole body. It was, apparently, Anaxagoras who first conceived some sort of a separation between mind and matter, but his notions were vague. Whereas his predecessors had imagined that we could only perceive things by having something within us which was like them, he held that we perceive in virtue of the presence within us of something opposed to the thing perceived.

Q

Mind or intelligence was for him an organizing and motive force, being simple and infinite as opposed to the complexity and limitation of matter over which it had power.

When we reach Aristotle we get ideas which smack of modern views, perhaps because we owe them to him. Matter, for him, was the substratum or continuant in Mr W. E. Johnson's sense ; whilst the form (eidos) made this matter a particular or determinate thing, and could be regarded as the soul of the thing. Now there was nothing essentially mental in this idea of a soul ; since every real thing animate or inanimate was possessed of a form. When dealing with organized matter this conception of a form corresponds to what would nowadays be regarded as its potential function. Thus, suppose the eye were an independent organism living apart from the body, its form would be the faculty of vision. The form or essence of the eye is its function of seeing, and we may say that the soul is to the body as a living whole or organism what vision is to the eye. In this sense there is nothing material or even mental about the soul, since its entire being is, in modern phraseology, functional. Such organization as the body possesses is entirely due to the soul. Body and soul thus mutually imply one another ; are correlatives : and it is a blunder to regard the soul as inhabiting a body in the sense that it could conceivably depart from it and take up its abode in another body. This would be about as reasonable as the assumption that vision could abandon the eye and go to dwell in the stomach.

In some such way as this Aristotle arrived at three kinds of souls which correspond to three forms of life ; the vegetative, the animal and the human. The soul of plants corresponds to the phenomena of nutrition and reproduction, for these are their functions. Animal souls are sensitive and appetitive, since sensations and locomotion are the functions of the animal body ; whilst human souls are characterized by reason or intelligence. The rational soul of human beings comprises within it, and unifies, the two inferior functions of nutrition and sensation. Thus it is evident that the soul was regarded not as something independent of the body but an immanent influence without which there could be neither unity nor bodily organization. Aristotle's conception of the mind is therefore what we should now name purely biological, though it differed from modern biology in acknowledging final causes.

So far all is plain, and, if not exactly intelligible, at all events the views are founded on direct facts of observation. Now there enters the villain of the piece in the shape of Descartes. He performed a veritable surgical operation by sharply cutting in two what had never before been so completely severed ; and thus at one blow rendered the science of physiology possible and confused the subject-matter of psychology. This deed was performed at the end of his sixth *Meditation* (3), thus, " Since, on the one hand, I have a clear and distinct idea of myself, in so far as I am only a thinking and unextended thing, and as, on the other hand I possess a distinct idea of body, in so far as it is only an extended and unthinking thing, it is certain that I, that is my mind, by which I am what I am, is entirely and truly distinct from my body and may exist without it." We may note that this astounding declaration is not founded on any facts of observation but purely on logical or epistemological grounds. It will be easily seen that on this view of body, what essentially distinguishes one portion of matter from another is the amount of extension in it. That is to say, matter consists of units whose sole characteristic is to be units ; or in other words it has no ultimate qualities except quantity. The essence of a nerve is the same as that of a stone ; both consist of quantitative units of extension. Of course there can be no relation of mind to matter on such a theory.

If we are to rely, however, on what is clear and distinct to the eye of reason then it was equally clear to Spinoza that to the eye of reason the whole of existence is interrelated, forming one all-embracing individuality ; and so, extension and thought were not for him distinct substances but attributes of one and the same substance. Thus both thought and extension, or if we prefer mind and matter, were equally real and stood, as it were, on the same plane. But Leibniz turned matter out of the universe because he could not form a clear notion of

an extended and unthinking thing. " Thus the world is not
a machine as Descartes and Hobbes would have it. Everything
in it is force, soul, life, thought, desire ; what we see is the
machine, but we only see the outside of Being. Being is that
which itself sees." The wheel has come full circle and we are
back again to a denial of the distinction between mind and
matter.

But this denial of dualism as a metaphysical theory does
not settle the question, since it is necessary to account for those
appearances which have led men to think that there are two
independent ultimate substances. How then are we to conceive
of them as related to each other ? For Aristotle the question
could not have arisen, since matter is the thing as it exists
potentially and form is the realization or actualization of this
potentiality. Matter is thus a mere naked possibility which
becomes a reality only when it is energized by form. And the
form has no existence apart from the matter of which it is
the realization. It never occurred to him to connect the brain
with thought, but had he done so he would probably have
said that we do not remember because we have a brain, but
we have a brain because we remember ; for he did say that
a man does not think because he has hands, he has hands
because he thinks. Whenever matter is met with, *i.e.* whenever
it is an actuality, as opposed to a mere potentiality, it carries
its form with it. The union of the soul with the body is but
a particular case of the unity of matter and form ; the soul
is the form of the body. In brief, soul and body, like form
and matter are correlative terms, logically distinguishable but
actually inseparable. " The soul can neither be without the
body, nor be itself a body of any kind, for it is not a body
but is yet something of the body and, therefore, present
innately in the body, and in a body peculiarly constituted."
It follows logically from this that all our activity is both
physical and psychical. Thus when a man is angry his emotion
has both a bodily and a mental aspect ; from the latter point
of view it is the desire to injure the man who has hurt him,
from the former it is the disturbance in the heart and other
organs. The curious may find in this view an anticipation

of the James-Lange theory of the emotions. Aristotle intended all this to apply, without reservation, only to the two inferior souls named above, but not to the human soul in its entirety.

With regard to this rational soul he drew a distinction between the active intellect and the passive intellect. (4) It is very difficult to understand what he meant by this distinction. He says " There must be within the soul a distinction answering to the general distinction between the matter which underlies each class of things and is potentially each of them, and the efficient cause which makes them—the distinction of which that between an art and its material is an instance." If we try to extract the meaning of this statement from the given analogy, it seems that art makes its objects by turning the material into objects fitted for artistic appreciation. Just as light converts colours which are potential into actual colours. Now we cannot identify the material here referred to with sense given material, since sense-data are the material of the sensitive or animal souls. Probably what Aristotle was trying to say was that the material presented to the active by the passive intellect was of the nature of propositions, and that the function of the active reason was to lick these into logical shape. Just as the animal soul has to work up the sense-data into sensible forms or percepts, so the active intellect has to work up the crude material of propositions into such as are amenable to logical judgment. (5)

Whether he meant this or not, it is quite clear that we ought to draw a distinction between the bare apprehension of propositions and the judgment passed upon them. The former is relatively passive and the latter active by comparison with it. If we regard the passive intellect as presenting material to the active it is possible to regard the former, like the lower faculties of sensation and imagination as entirely dependent on the body. It would, therefore, perish with the body. Not so the active intellect ; which being comparable to the subject in the subject-object relation persists by its own right. The active intellect is a vital and imperishable principle, separable from the passive and not, therefore, subject to the limitations of time and circumstance to which the latter is bound. To such a theory psychology has nothing to say, and there can never be any evidence of a factual kind to discredit it. It is obviously a theological and metaphysical doctrine to be tested by the facts and canons to which these studies have reference. We may, however, say that no evidence from the psychological sphere of facts can invalidate it. The question of the immortality of the soul is to this extent outside the realm of psychological and, I may add, physical considerations.

When Descartes had sundered matter and mind, by limiting the one to extension and the other to thought, he then proceeded to the relation of body to mind, which he was aware was a different problem altogether. On his mechanical principle the body, being an automatic machine, had all the motive force necessary to move it in itself, just as a wound clock needs no external source of energy. But he seems to have thought that, since the mind obviously did act on the body, it could do so by changing the direction of the motion of the animal spirits, but not the quantity of the motion. Still he was perfectly well aware that all such analogies broke down in the unique case presented by the mind-body problem. He, therefore, threw up the sponge and, on true Bergsonian lines, he asserted that the only way of understanding the relation was to live through it. *Solvitur ambulando.* " That the mind, which is incorporeal, is able to move the body, we know neither by reasoning nor by any comparison with other things ; nevertheless, we cannot doubt it, since we are too clearly informed of it by experiences which are too certain and too evident. And we must keep in mind that this is one of those things that are known by themselves, and that we render these more obscure whenever we try to explain them by other things." It would have saved a good deal of controversy if philosophers had remembered that, on Cartesian principles, there can be no relation between matter and mind, whilst Descartes himself believed that there could be no separation between mind and body. The importance of the distinction justifies another quotation from his sixth *Meditation.* " Nature, likewise, teaches us by sensations of pain, hunger, thirst, etc., that *I am not only lodged in my body as a pilot in a vessel, but that I am besides so intimately conjoined, and, as it were, intermixed with it that my mind and body compose a certain unity* (italics mine). For if this were not the case, I should not feel pain when my body is hurt, seeing I am merely a thinking thing, but should perceive the wound by the understanding alone, just as a pilot perceives by sight when any part of his vessel is damaged." It is perfectly clear that on this topic Descartes repudiated the Cartesian philosophy, or, if he did not, that he perceived clearly that the union of mind and body was a unity *sui generis.*

The perplexities in which philosophers have been involved are due to the tacit assumption, previously mentioned, that the relation of body to mind is the same as the relation of matter to mind ; or, to put it in a slightly different way, that there is no difference in relationship between a mind and its body and the same mind and foreign bodies. But this is so palpably absurd that it is hard to see how anyone could ever have imagined it. If I wish to move my arm I do so immediately and there is nothing, that I am aware of, that intervenes between the volition and the movement. If it is said that a series of nervous impulses must travel down the brachial nerves before this can be accomplished, the statement is correct but quite misleading. For, of such impulses I know nothing until the physiologist enlightens me. Neither in perception nor in volition have I ever any direct knowledge of brain processes of any sort. (6) My brain and my nerves are completely diaphanous as far as my perceptions and actions are concerned. Most human beings, like Aristotle, have lived out their lives without being aware that there was any relation between mind and brain ; and all of us would do so unless physiologists and psychologists had told us otherwise.

It may be objected that in cases of paralysis a man may desire to move his arm and yet be unable to do so ; and that, therefore, the relation is not direct. But we have seen that, in cases of hemiplegia, the ability is only temporary and that an emotion or strong volition will bring about the movement, even in those cases where the assumed necessary part of the brain is missing. If the brachial nerve is completely severed of course I shall not be able to move my arm, but then my arm is no longer part of my body—it is just as much a foreign body as the arm of someone else.

As long as my body is animated by my mind so long is my relation to it different from my relation to all other bodies, animated or not. The relation is so intimate, the *rapport* is so close that it is only by analogies that it can be described, for it cannot be reduced to simpler terms. William James (7) thought otherwise. " Between what a man calls *me* and what he calls *mine*," he said, " the line is difficult to draw. We feel and act about certain things that are ours very much as we feel and act about ourselves. . . . *In its widest sense a man's Me is the sum total of all that he can call his*, not only his body and his psychic powers, but his clothes and his house, his wife and children, his ancestors and friends, his reputation and his works, his lands and his horses, and yacht and bank-account. All these things give him the same emotions. If they wax and prosper, he feels triumphant ; if they dwindle and die away, he feels cast down,—not necessarily in the same degree for each thing, but in much the same way for all."

This eloquent description does violence to the facts, by picturesquely lumping the body together with a strange assortment of associates, and affirming that they all have the same relation to the mind. If somebody beats my children or tears my clothes I shall feel hurt, but I shall feel hurt in a totally different sense if he batters my face or tears my skin. And not all the eloquence in the world can reduce the difference in my feelings to a difference of degree. If James had made use of a different collection of instances he would have come nearer to the heart of the matter. He ought to have considered the relation of the instruments or tools that a man uses to accomplish his purposes to the man himself. A youth begins to learn to ride a bicycle, let us say. At first it is quite out of his control and does nothing that he desires. It is completely a foreign body as far as he is concerned. Let him but persist and go on using it, and eventually he acquires perfect control over it : and for purposes of getting about it becomes almost part of him, If he could only derive sensations from it, as he almost does after years of use, it might be considered an organ, like his legs. The same is true of any other instrument or tool that a man uses to accomplish his purposes. Thus a blind man gropes his way with a stick, and when he probes the ground what he feels is, not the stick, but the parts of the ground he is exploring. The stick is almost, but, of course, not quite, like our nervous system in being diaphanous ; it is in fact almost like an elongated finger. The *rapport* is more immediate when we use an organ like the eye ; for when I look at a landscape I do not perceive my eye, in any sense of the term, but the scene alone. The relation of the body to the mind is more intimate and direct than the relation of any instrument that may be used ; it is the functional relation *par excellence.*

A wonderful series of movements is made by the tongue in changing the shape of the mouth cavity to produce sounds. But nobody, except the trained phonetician, can discriminate these movements. For the rest of us the mere thought of uttering the words is sufficient to bring about the necessary speech movements. In learning to speak a foreign tongue by the aid of phonetic charts the movements are laboriously made until we have acquired the necessary skill, when we cease to be conscious of them, just as happens in the case of learning to ride a bicycle. Still, however close the analogy, no instrument ever does come to bear the same relation to our activities that the organism does. The difference is shewn by a fact that is so trivial as hardly to be worth pointing out, namely that I feel a sensation of pain when one of my organs functions badly but only annoyance when my pen or any other instrument refuses to function satisfactorily. If, by some miracle, my pen were to grow into my hand after years of use, no doubt I should feel a prick of pain when the nib began to splutter. However that may be, in the organic world function always determines structure as we saw when dealing with the bodily mechanisms which are supposed to underlie instinctive actions. And it is because Aristotle recognized this functional relation that his views are still of importance in the mind-body problem.

A disembodied mind could not act on matter nor receive

impressions from without.   Nor could material things be related to such a mind, whatever the believers in telepathy may say to the contrary.   Such views, when held by philosophers, form a striking example of the ability to hold opinions which are in direct conflict with one another.   Only a mind-body can affect the material world outside it or be affected by it.   A ghost and a corpse are strange bed-fellows fit only to generate savage theories ; whereas an animated body is not two things, but one organized whole.   There is nothing, therefore, strange in supposing that the parts of this whole must be in direct *rapport* with each other, and this is the view we shall develop later.

Spinoza avoided this blunder, as he clearly saw that, on Cartesian principles, there could be no relation between mind and matter ; and he rightly asked what clear conception Descartes could have of thought intimately connected with a portion of matter.   And he objected to the latter calling in God to help him out of his metaphysical difficulty.   Spinoza maintained that thinking substance and material substance were one and the same, regarded from different standpoints.   Consequently, since nobody can deny that animals are animated, it must follow that all the universe is animated in a greater or less degree.   The kind of relation that subsists between body and mind is accordingly but a particular case of the general relation of mind to matter.   There is an apparent parallelism between bodily and mental attributes due to the underlying identity of substance.   " The mind and the body are one and the same thing, conceived at one time under the attribute of thought, and at another time under that of extension.   For this reason the order and concatenation of things is one whether nature be conceived under this or that attribute, and consequently the order of the actions and passions of our body is coincident in nature with the order of the actions and passions of the mind."   Unless we adopt this standpoint on general metaphysical grounds, and regard the universe as spiritually animated through and through, the two problems of matter and mind and of mind and body throw no light upon each other.

It is very interesting to observe that two recent philosophers, Professor S. Alexander and Mr C. Lloyd Morgan hold somewhat similar views. The latter, in fact, is an avowed adherent of Spinoza. He thinks that life emerged during the course of evolution, when matter had attained a certain stage of complexity ; and that at a later stage of complexity mind emerged from living matter. (8) This doctrine of emergent evolution insists that the new qualities which emerge have new relations which are not predictable in any sense from the old relations. With emergence new features come into existence. But, lest anyone should think that mind emerges from the void, Mr Lloyd Morgan is careful to insist that, from the primordial stuff out of which matter is composed right up through the various steps of evolution, " every natural entity, from atom to man expresses both attributes," physical and psychical.

Philosophers have a passion for a unified universe and can only understand it if they detect the principle of unity. Spinoza started from a world-soul, which was the principle of unity for him, and worked down to the mind-body problem as a particular instance of it. Leibniz worked the other way round. His starting point was the mind-body relation and in this way he attempted to account for the unity of the universe. In opposition to the Cartesian view of matter as a quantitative inert thing, his conception of matter was derived from the concept of an organism. (9) Only if all parts of the universe were organically related could there be any real connection between them. Thus the real elements of material things were not inert atoms, but each had a certain power or spontaneity which alone made them real things, as opposed to the abstractions of physical science. We may get a clearer view of what he meant by considering the views of modern biologists on the nature of the development of growing organisms.

The fertilized egg-cell of the sea urchin and other forms, like all other fertilized ova proceeds, under suitable conditions, to divide into two cells. Each of these cells gives rise to one-half of the body, one to the right half, the other to the left. But, if the cells are separated, each eventually produces a complete individual, *i.e.* the cell which would have produced a right half produces the whole, and similarly with the cell which would have produced the left half. It is obvious that both cells have the potentiality to produce a whole individual, but what each does produce is dependent on its relation to the other. This relation persists when the cells further divide, and has been shewn to hold true for a large number of animals where observation is possible, such as the Amphibia. When, by constant division, a hollow spherical mass of cells is produced certain definite portions gives rise to the brain, others to the eyes, the alimentary canal and so forth. It looks as though all is predetermined in the growing egg. But this is an error. For, if from the region that is to produce the skin (say) a part is removed and transplanted to the region where the brain is in course of being developed, the fate of the transplanted cells is changed and they produce brain material instead of skin. That is to say the development takes such a course as to produce structures which are fitted to the position in which they find themselves. Any individual cell can therefore take part in the production of a great variety of tissues, depending on its relation to such tissues.

As Professor H. S. Jennings (10) has summed it up : " What a cell becomes, what line of development it follows, depends, not merely on what it has within it, but on its relation to the other cells. . . . The cells adapt themselves and their developmental processes to the conditions in the cells that constitute their immediate environment. Thus from the beginning development is adjustment to the environment ; adjustment of parts to each other. . . . The fate of the cells, in these early stages, is determined, not by different genes [parts of the nuclei] contained in different cells [for each cell contains all the genes] ; not even, in the main, by the diverse cytoplasm contained in different cells, but by the conditions surrounding each cell. The same set of genes produces different things, follows a different course of action, under different surrounding conditions. This is the great and important fact which emerges from the study of early development." It thus appears that though the potentiality of a particular mode of life exists in each cell its actuality depends on the working out of the potentialities of all the other cells in its cellular environment. Of course the farther away any particular cell is from some particular tissue the less will the influence be.

Now let us follow the clue suggested by these facts of organic development, and as we are now dealing with ultimate philosophical matters let us allow our fancy to roam. Suppose we have traced the growth of the fertilized ovum until it has reached the stage of the gastrula, a spherical mass of cells. We may, for the purposes of analogy, regard this mass as a microcosm of the world we are trying to understand. Each cell may be compared to one of the real units of the universe, a Leibnizian monad. (9) Every such monad has within it the potentialities of the whole macrocosm just as each cell is a potential animal. It, therefore, in some way, reflects the constitution of the whole universe. It has, as Leibniz would have said, a ' perception ' of the whole, *i.e.* it represents the whole in an ideal form. But, in addition, each monad has a certain spontaneity, just as our cells have a power of self-production, *i.e.* it has ' appetition.' It is in virtue of its appetition that the monad is able to unfold spontaneously all the potentiality of that which it represents.

Monads, each possessing the qualities of perception and appetition are the metaphysical units out of which the universe is constructed. Perception and appetition in the monad are unconscious ; but conscious perception and conscious striving are the distinguishing characters of mind. Hence the monads are primitive minds or souls. Each monad pursues its own course of self-development, but as each reflects the whole world from its own point of view, and as the whole is potentially contained in each, they are all in harmony. Instead of our harmonious series of cells working to a common goal Leibniz used the analogy of a number of independent choirs, which pay no attention to one another and yet keep in unison because they are all singing from the same piece of music. But why do all our cells in the growing organism work in unison to the production of an animal body ? That, according to this view, is because they have had the harmony impressed

upon them by the Creator. The soul and body are two such
collections of monads : " The soul follows its own laws, and
the body likewise follows its laws ; and they agree with each
other in virtue of the pre-established harmony between all
substances, since they are representations of one and the
same universe." By this system of monadology Leibniz
attempted to reduce our two problems to one ; the relation
of mind to matter being but an instance of the relation of mind
to body. But we see that this is only accomplished by calling
in the help of God, the great harmonizer of the universe to
whom all monads must submit though they follow their own
individual development.

The parts of the organism, including of course the nervous
system, are a society of subordinate monads, standing, however,
to the dominant monad, the soul, in a peculiarly intimate
relation. Just as a society of persons formed for some particular purpose, such as the members of a college, are for this
purpose in much closer *rapport* with each other than they are
with those outside the society. The relationship subsisting
between a society of persons is different from that subsisting
between any other collection of individual things. It was for
this reason that James Ward, who favoured Leibniz' position,
called the relation between the mind and its body an inter-
subjective relation in contrast with the foreign or objective
relations which prevailed between this body and anything
outside it. (6) When we remember that one of the greatest
contributions made by Ward to the science of psychology was
to emphasize the universality of the subject-object relation
in mental events, to call the relation of mind to body an
inter-subjective relation is equivalent to the denial that the
body is related to the mind as other bodies are related to it.
The relation is similar to that which would exist if two minds
were telepathically related to each other, so as to communicate
without any intervening medium.

What it all comes to is this. When we consider a living
body we have no right to assume that its functions are in any
sense those of a non-living body. All statements to the
contrary made by biologists are simply due to the fact that

they are under the impression that the only real things in the universe are electrons and protons, and that the nature of these is known to the physicists. But this, as we shall see later, is a soulless blunder. The brain, as a part of my anatomy, studied as it appears to a physiologist, is a totally different thing from the brain when it carries out my purposes. When I am dead my brain as examined by a physiologist has exactly the same fibres and arrangements as it had when I was alive. The physiologist is, therefore, deceived into believing that he is somehow studying the brain as an organ of the mind. But this, of course, he cannot do. His relation to my brain is an objective or foreign relation ; and the only brain to which he has any other relation, the mind-body relation, is his own ; which he is for ever precluded from studying. If by an ingenious arrangement of X-ray photography on the television principle he could observe his own brain, as he observes mine, his relation to his own brain, for that particular observation, would be a purely objective or foreign relation. He can never get inside his own brain subjectively from an objective stand-point. Thus he is for ever precluded from studying the mind-problem by any other than a psychological or philosophical method of approach.

By this time the reader will have had enough of it. He will say what have all these far-fetched analogies and subtle distinctions to do with either of the problems under consideration ? The mind is not the brain and the former is mental, the latter material. How can they possibly be related ? Well ; that is the problem which these distinctions are intended to elucidate. If we are steeped in mechanical views of the nature of matter, regarding atoms as little hard balls it is irritating to be told that a portion of matter is a colony of minds. Let us then turn to the physical sciences and ask how they describe the same piece of material. This will soften the blow and make us less irritable. Physicists have been no less revolutionary in their treatment of matter than philosophers and we had better see what they make of it, and more especially whether they consider its nature to be inorganic.

We have learnt that Descartes, thinking that he had a clear

idea of extended matter, sundered matter from mind, only to join the two again when it was a question of body and mind. Now the first thing that modern physics has done is to deny that we have clear ideas of extension, and further to emphasize the fact that any idea of extension that we may have does not apply to the ultimate parts of matter. Extension being composed of lengths and areas is entirely relative to the standpoint of the observer ; and matter is as empty as anything can be. In fact Professor Eddington has estimated that if we collected all ultimate constituents in a man's body into one heap the resulting mass would be a speck just visible with a magnifying glass ; all the rest is empty space. (11) Leaving the empty space aside, matter is composed of two sorts of units, with opposite electric charges, namely protons and electrons, all of which are exactly alike as far as their properties are concerned. Instead of a colony of unextended minds, all mirroring the universe from their own standpoints, a piece of matter is a colony of atoms, consisting of planetary systems, each mirroring the universe but having no fixed standpoint from which to do it. An atom consists of a nucleus made of a proton, or a proton and electrons, around which electrons are scattered in various fixed orbits ; but any one can escape and wander through the material. But this is not the worst that physics has done to matter. So far we might be tempted to substitute for the original hard billiard-ball-like atoms of the old chemistry equally definite electrons and protons. This, however, we are not allowed to do. For the only thing that physicists tell us about these units is that they are sources of radiations or waves which are capable of mathematical treatment.

Certain experimental observations on the electron shew that it produces effects similar to the interference and diffraction of light. Whence it is inferred that an electron, like light, must be considered as being something of the nature of waves. The physics of the electron is fast becoming wave mechanics, for as Professor Eddington (11) says : " The equations for the motion of the wave-group with given frequency and potential frequency are the same as the classical equations of the motion of a particle with the corresponding energy and potential energy." But waves are something which we can picture, and even experience when we are at sea ; and lest there should be any trace of the old material 'matter' surviving, these waves which constitute the electron are assigned to a sub-æther which is outside the range of any possible sensory experience. " The entity which we suppose to be oscillating when we speak of the waves in the sub-æther . . . is denoted by ψ, and properly speaking we should regard it as an elementary indefinable of the wave theory. But can we give it a classical interpretation of any kind ? It seems possible to interpret it as a probability. The probability of the particle or electron being within a given region is proportional to the amount of ψ in that region . . . and there is no definite localization of the electron, though some places are more probable than others." But suppose, by some miracle, we were able to hit on the exact position of an electron we should still be no better off ; for it is believed that, when dealing with microscopic quantities such as an electron, we can only attain to a knowledge of its position by foregoing a knowledge of its velocity. It is very refreshing, after demolishing all traces of gross material substance and replacing it by a series of waves existing we know not where, to learn that in Professor Eddington's view wave-mechanics is not a physical theory, but an ingenious dodge for representing by symbols something of which we can never have any direct knowledge.

Knowing nothing about the nature of the centre from which the waves emanate, not even where the centre is situated, but knowing a good deal about the mathematical symbols by which waves are interpreted, physics substitutes these symbols for 'matter.' As Mr Bertrand Russell (12) has wittily expressed it : " When energy radiates from a centre, we can describe the laws of its radiation conveniently by imagining something in the centre, which we will call an electron or a proton according to circumstances, and for certain purposes it is convenient to regard this centre as persisting, *i.e.* as not a single point in space-time but a series of such points, separated

R

from each other by time-like intervals. All this, however, is only a convenient way of describing what happens elsewhere, namely the radiation of energy away from the centre. As to what goes on in the centre itself, if anything, physics is silent. . . . 'Matter' is convenient formula for describing what happens where it isn't. I am talking physics, not metaphysics." This seems to be an error, for in view of what has been said above he appears to be talking mathematics, *i.e.* describing the nature of symbols instead of the nature of matter. But in all probability that is as near as the new physics ever can get in dealing with the nature of matter on physical lines.

But although the study of symbolic expressions is a task worthy of a philosopher we must not be misled into supposing that the mathematical interpretation of matter is the only valid one. The experimental facts, or the concepts by which they are interpreted, can be regarded from a totally different standpoint. We are in fact witnessing a revival of what happened in the seventeenth century. Physics made rapid strides then, and the physical concepts of that age dominated future thinking. As Professor A. N. Whitehead (13) has pointed out these concepts were quite unsuitable to the biological sciences, and when taken over by physiologists introduced insoluble problems into the study of organisms and life. This is happening again. The success of physical science and its prestige make biologists and psychologists very ready to accept the concepts derived from this study, in the hope that their own studies may become truly scientific. On the principle of explaining the unknown by the known they attempt to use physical ideas to explain life. " The appeal to mechanism on behalf of biology [and psychology] was in its origin an appeal to the well attested self-consistent physical concepts as expressing the basis of all material phenomena. But at present there is no such system of concepts. Science is taking on a new aspect which is neither purely physical, nor purely biological. It is becoming the study of organisms. Biology is the study of the larger organisms ; whereas physics is the study of the smaller organisms."

At last the wheel has come full circle again and the constitution of matter as a colony of organisms is no longer absurd but has high philosophic and physical sanction. What we now have to do is to revise our notions of matter so as to make them harmonize with our ideas of organism, instead of interpreting our ideas of organic life in terms of matter. This is what Professor Whitehead has attempted to do, and thereby to rectify the wrong ideas that have crept into our thinking as the result of the discoveries of the seventeenth century. His point of departure is constituted by the fact that the atom is a vibratory system radiating energy. It is not a bare collection of isolated electrons and protons but a systematic whole. The organization of the whole as a system of interconnected events is the true reality ; whereas the isolated electrons considered as independently enduring and unchanging particles are mere abstractions. Reality is an organized system. Thus living bodies are not differentiated from others by the fact of being organized, since all are organisms. This conception is a great advance on all previous ideas, and in particular avoids the necessity of assuming the pre-established harmony which Leibniz was compelled to postulate in order to get his colony of monads to function organically.

Another great advantage of this organic view is that our two problems of matter and mind and mind and body are once again reduced to one. For an organic plan has reference to a whole system of events and has no significance apart from a system. Hence, as Whitehead says (13), " In the case of an animal, the mental states enter into the plan of the total organism and thus modify the plans of the successive subordinate organisms until the smallest organisms, such as electrons, are reached. Thus an electron within a living body is different from an electron outside it, by reason of the plan of the body. The electron blindly runs either within or without the body ; but it runs within the body in accordance with its character within the body ; that is to say, in accordance with the general plan of the body, and this plan includes the mental state. But the principle of modification is perfectly general throughout nature, and represents no property peculiar to living bodies."

This is the acutest thing said about the mind-body problem since the time of Aristotle. If I interpret it correctly it means that we can never learn anything about the mind from a study of the brain alone ; and up to the present this has been strictly verified by experience. Nevertheless this view, which reduces our two problems to one, is not completely satisfactory in that it places mind and body in the same category of ultimate realities.

The view which we shall develop in the next chapter, and which our whole argument in this book has suggested, is that mind and matter are in different categories. According to Professor Eddington all that physics ever can discover about matter is a system of differential equations and not what is behind these. In fact what is behind them is a question of no importance or relevance to physics. We derive our knowledge of matter by means of measuring instruments, and the subject matter of physics is the reading of such instruments. Force, activity, energy and everything else that the physicist deals with have only a logical significance within a realm of instrumental observations. They form a closed system within which the mind does not enter but which it simply contemplates and reduces to order. The one thing we are certain of is that no substance or ' matter ' binds the whole together. But not a single feature of this is true of mind. A knowledge of that does not rest on readings of instruments, or on external observation, or on inference. We know the facts of mind by living through them, by subjective experience. We have, in other words, direct insight in this realm, as opposed to inferential knowledge in the other.

CHAPTER XII

MIND AND BODY

Now that the physical world has been shattered into symbols only cemented together by differential equations we may approach the mind-body problem without too many misconceptions. When Dr Johnson struck his foot against a large stone, in order to refute Berkeley's idealistic philosophy, and rebounded from it, he little thought that he was kicking a collection of waves or symbols. He was too matter-of-fact a person to be a philosopher, but the tingling sensation of pain in his toe, which it is to be presumed he received, ought to have convinced him that some part, at least, of the sensations he derived from the stone were not there but in his mind.

The traditional theories about the relation of mind to body, namely psycho-physical parallelism and interactionism have always proceeded on three erroneous assumptions. The first is that the epistemology derived from the study of natural science must hold for this particular relation. Thus interaction is assumed to be intelligible only if the kind of action we have in mind is that guaranteed by physics. But physics nowadays no longer assumes as axiomatic that action amongst electrons must be of the same kind as action between large sensible bodies. The macroscopic epistemology is cheerfully cast away when dealing with microscopic action, and nobody winces at the contradiction. If, therefore, anybody can suggest a new type of action when body and mind interact there is nothing to prevent him doing so. He need not search in the macroscopic physical world for action of a like kind, since we have seen, in an earlier chapter, that mental activity is *toto coelo* different from physical. As the world contemplated by natural science is a symbolic world there is obviously one kind of relation easily possible between it and the mind, the relation of knowing. And this relation is obviously peculiar to this one set of terms. Whatever view we take of the nature of mind it alone can know symbols and manipulate them. Similarly there is nothing in current epistemology which prevents us from asserting that the instrumental relation between body and mind need not follow the analogy of the instrumental relation current in the physical world. It may be an instrumental relation *sui generis*. That is, when we speak of the body being the instrument by which the mind accomplishes its purposes, we must not expect that the instrument is of the kind we are familiar with when physical purposes are accomplished.

The second assumption is that the living body is an entity of the same kind as inanimate bodies. If Professor Whitehead's view is correct, namely, that all inanimate bodies are of the nature of organisms, no objection can be taken to this assumption. But if it is meant that the properties of living bodies are the same as those of inanimate bodies it is palpably wrong. Let us consider the properties of nervous tissue, which is assumed to be in a more intimate relation with the mind than any other tissue. We know that nerve fibres obey the " all-or-none " law in response to electrical stimulation, but this is a property of living nerve and there is nothing comparable to it in a dead piece of tissue. Again the wave of negative potential which passes down a nerve fibre on being stimulated is a peculiar property of living nerves unlike anything in a dead piece of tissue ; and the latter on being stimulated would, presumably, pass a wave of positive potential. And there is one feature of living sensory nerves which is not only not matched in anything else, but which is inconceivable even as a possibility ; namely, that any stimulus to an afferent nerve trunk ultimately yields a sensation. What is the sense, then, of shutting our eyes to these differences and refusing to regard the living as totally distinct from the inanimate ? When considering the relation of mind to body we ought obviously only to mean the relation to the living body.

It was said above that the mind is supposed to be in some peculiar way more attached to the nerve impulses, and to such impulses in one particular region, than to any other living process. This is the third of the assumptions underlying the hypotheses of parallelism and interactionism and is worthy of close consideration. We are here dealing with one of the most firmly held dogmas of physiological psychology, namely that consciousness is intimately associated with the cerebral cortex ; that in fact, the latter is, in some way, the organ of mind. Or, if that is expressed in too materialistic terms, it is thought that the mind and the brain are functionally related in some more intimate sense than that in which the rest of the body is related to consciousness. Professor G. F. Stout (1) states the matter very clearly. After describing how sensory impulses are conveyed from the sense organ to the cortex and efferent impulses are sent thence to the muscular system, he proceeds thus : " We may notice at the outset that if the circuit be interrupted, say by a section of the nerves, at any point before the impulse reaches the cerebral hemispheres, the conscious process fails to arise. . . . It is thus natural to suppose that normal consciousness is only directly connected with the central phases of the process. On a variety of grounds we are justified in thinking that nothing which takes place in other parts of the nervous system is found to make any difference to consciousness except in so far as it gives rise to changes in the cerebral cortex and its annex the midbrain ; on the other hand, the suspension or alteration of certain cerebral processes appears uniformly to be accompanied by suspension or alteration of conscious process. Hence we may conclude generally that in the cerebral cortex alone, the mental life of which we are normally conscious is directly conditioned by neural occurrences. This general doctrine is further defined and confirmed by the results of investigation into the localization of cerebral functions."

We have already seen that the whole doctrine of the localization of function is invalid, so that nothing more need be said about this confirmation of the belief that consciousness is in a direct way conditioned by the cortex. All the other arguments ever brought forward to substantiate the view that the cerebrum is the seat of consciousness rest on erroneous views as to the nature of organic life. They all assume that the parts of the organism can act in isolation just as they act when organically united ; that, in fact, an organism is a bare summation of organs, just as a machine consists of separate parts each of which can be used for other machines. But the outstanding characteristic of organisms is the interdependence of each organ on the proper functioning of all the other organs. To suppose that the liver, for example, could function without the heart to give it a proper blood supply is absurd ; and so of all the other organs in the body. Cut out the kidneys and sooner or later all the other organs, including the nervous system, cease to function. Does a bad digestion make no difference to consciousness ? If so, then what becomes of the doctrine of temperament as affected by the bodily constitution ? Let us try cutting out the lungs. The circuit is then also broken and consciousness ceases. If this is too drastic, we may try cutting off the air supply. But consciousness then ceases too. In the same sense in which consciousness is said to be conditioned by nervous processes it is also conditioned by any other vital process, and by the essential parts of the environment. Any other view of the relation of consciousness to the body is founded upon unjustified abstractions, and not upon real vital processes. Even if we confine ourselves to the abstraction of isolated nervous impulses there is still no ground for thinking that what goes on in the cortex is more important or direct for conscious life than what goes on elsewhere.

For, as the behaviourists have insisted, and this is their sole merit as psychologists though they are excellent physiologists, consciousness is accompanied by changes macroscopic and microscopic in the remotest parts of the body system. The real business in a telephone system is not done by the telephone girls, who merely plug in and plug out, but by the subscribers at the end of the receivers. If ever any light is thrown on the mystery of consciousness from the bodily side (and this we have seen good reason to doubt) it will come from the consideration of what general conditions constitute vital processes as distinguished from lifeless ones. And, apart from the behaviouristic bias, I am in agreement with Mr J. F.

Dashiell (2) when he says : " Introspective descriptions made by the man who does the thinking, tally distinctly better with the conception of the business as one that goes on in the large regions of the body, rather than in a temporarily sealed-up cerebrum. Thinking thus becomes in a true sense a matter of a man's actually adjusting himself and his doings. To hold that the brain is the one principal and important locus of the thinking mechanism in a very peculiar and special way is a wholly gratuitous assumption." This opinion, at any rate, is much more in accordance with sound biological thinking than the view that nervous impulses can be isolated from the rest of organic life, or that they play some mysterious rôle not shared by other vital processes in determining consciousness. The artificiality of the separation of the brain from the rest of the body provides one explanation of why no light has ever been thrown on the mind-body problem by the study of the nervous system. We have been searching in one corner for something which is only intelligible when we consider the organism as a whole, and the relations of its various parts. Just like the American lady, who, having visited the Bank of England, asked the policeman outside to direct her to the Church of England.

We may go a stage further than this and refuse to consider that the organism has any meaning apart from its environment. As it is an artificial abstraction to separate one organ from another so it is equally artificial to attempt to separate the organism as a whole from its environment. This is a commonplace of biology ; and has been forcibly expressed by Mr A. D. Ritchie (2) with whose whole general position I am in sympathy. He says : " The organism possesses a sort of core, the central nervous system, which is a system of events of a specially elaborate and highly integrated type. As we pass outwards from this core, we pass to simpler and less integrated sets of events until finally we reach a region where there is no sign of organisation that is related to the organisation of the core. Starting with events that constitute the brain, we pass from the centre of organic activities to those belonging to less and less essential parts of the body, then to what is mostly outside the body, and finally to what has no relevance at all to the life history of the organism. It is important to realise that to reach a region of events entirely irrelevant to the organism one has to go very far afield, in fact, outside the solar system."

A function presupposes both an organism and an environment and is unintelligible without them. Whenever marvellous tales are told about instincts springing up, fully equipped, as the result of maturation of the organism alone, we may be sure that we are dealing with incorrect observations or hasty deductions therefrom. Thus a chick's initial pecking at small objects, on emerging from the shell, has been shewn to be due to rapid learning ; and we must not forget that the chick has performed movements in the egg, pecking its way out. Even sex behaviour, which we might consider to be predetermined in the lower animals by the possession of suitable organs, shews remarkable abnormalities in animals raised under peculiar conditions and is dependent on a suitable environment. Mr L. Carmichael (3) hit upon the happy idea of drugging the eggs of frogs and salamanders, thus allowing them to mature without movements, and then comparing their subsequent swimming functions with those of normally reared eggs. He concluded that the mere maturation of the neuro-muscular system provided no explanation of its functions. There is no sudden outburst of function, but from the initial twitch to the fully co-ordinated swimming movements there is a continuum of increasingly complex responses. The swimming co-ordination is not perfect at the first trial. In other words the inheritance of an organ is dependent on the environment. A hereditary ' given ' is transformed by an environmental ' present ' and any separation of the two is an abstraction. The growth of any organism can only be understood in terms of continual living function. And even the growth of a particular organ, the maturation of its muscular and nervous mechanisms, is only intelligible if we remember that there is a continuous functional stimulation within the organism itself due to its particular cellular environment, which is, in its turn, in functional relation with the outside world. The upshot of the whole matter is what we cannot, in any intelligible sense, consider a function as associated only with a particular organ, and that an organ has no meaning apart from an environment. In particular, it is absurd to suppose that the functioning of the cerebral cortex is more directly connected with consciousness than any other organ. And, if there were any meaning in the phrase the ' localization of consciousness,' we should be forced to conclude that it is localized exactly where the organism and environment are localized, that is in the world at large.

The hypothesis of psycho-physical parallelism is a pure guess, very wide of the mark, and a roundabout way of stating the one-to-one correspondence between mind and body, which we shall consider below. It is based on an outworn physiology ; and the observations derived from cerebral injuries which we considered in an early chapter, and more especially the study of aphasia, shew that there is no factual evidence whatever for it. The only kind of parallelism which is worthy of serious consideration is that which considers the parallel events in mind and body so close as to be identical, namely the doctrine of Spinoza.

But although the doctrine finds no justification in the facts of physiology it is frequently supposed to be warranted on general philosophical grounds. And the two theories of parallelism and interactionism are held together ; the two sets of events mental and bodily are parallel, but they also react on each other. It is assumed, as axiomatic, that there must be a correspondence between structural and functional units of organization. This supposed correspondence must, it is thought, extend to the minutest portions of the nervous system, single cells specialized for definite functions. The mathematical bias of modern epistemology goes beyond this and seeks a correspondence in ultra microscopical units, whereby the ultimate elements of the physical world, electrons and protons must have a correspondence with the supposed ultimate units of consciousness. But the supposed mental units belong to an atomic psychology which has long since been abandoned. Nevertheless the prestige of mathematical epistemology is sufficiently great to justify a further examination of this assumed correspondence.

The most interesting and instructive example of the one-to-one correspondence between mind and body is that given by Professor Eddington (1). This is well worthy of close study on several grounds, the chief of which is the implied assumption that mental events are not intelligible unless we can point to some corresponding physical background, which in some way must reproduce them, point for point. The problem concerns the nature of Time as a physical entity. Professor Eddington has emphasized the fact that the primary laws of the physical world, *i.e.* the laws concerning individuals, can be stated without any reference to time. The only way in which time occurs in the mathematical statement of such laws is by positive and negative signs ; but these are arbitrary and can all be reversed without any significant change. Just as it makes no difference to the properties of a square, for example, if its sides are specified as plus or minus a certain length, so it makes no difference to the laws of motion if positive and negative times are interchanged. Time is *not* of the essence of the laws. Whether a particle has moved out from the past into the present or moves into the future is entirely irrelevant to the statement of the laws ; and it can even move, if it wishes to, from the future to the past without affecting the symbolic statement.

But there is one physical law, dealing not with individuals but with aggregates, which, according to Professor Eddington, does recognize a difference in direction in time, namely the second law of thermo-dynamics. With a touch of genius he attributes this necessity for taking into account the flow of time in physical events to the fact of organization. The increase of entropy, or the running down of energy from a more available to a less usable form, is the measure of the increasing disorganization which is going on in the world. So, a well ordered army can accomplish the purposes of a state, but it becomes less and less effective for such purposes the more disorganization sets in. Similarly the increase of entropy makes energy less available, and the universe is running down. As this change is irreversible, the statement of the second law is the symbolic representation of the fact that time is a directed quantity with a real past and a real future. This saves the situation ; for, not only is a world where nothing really happens an uncomfortable one to live in, but we are conscious of change ; and although it may be an illusion that we are growing different it is undoubtedly a fact that we are always growing older. Accordingly Professor Eddington maintains that something must be going on in the physical world, and since a symbolic representation of the world disguises this fact, therefore "Consciousness, looking out through a private door, can learn by direct insight an underlying character of the world which physical measures do not betray."

I believe this psychological belief to be a true statement of the case, and its further development is also psychologically unexceptionable, namely that : " We have direct insight into ' becoming ' which sweeps aside all symbolic knowledge as on an inferior plane. If I grasp the notion of existence because I myself exist, I grasp the notion of becoming because I myself become." Admirable ! It is beyond this point, however, that the psychological difficulty emerges. If the above argument is sound there really is a time direction in the physical world ; and we know on *perfectly independent* introspective psychological evidence that there is an immediate consciousness of time in the mental world ; though it does not follow that the latter is an accurate measure of the former. If it were there would be no use for clocks. It will be a convenience to have a separate term to express the consciousness of time *as it is felt*, and by analogy with such expressions as ' enduring a pain ' I shall call it endurance. Time, as immediately experienced, will be said to be endured.

Now Professor Eddington maintains that the mind not only perceives the passing of time in the world of physical events but also is immediately aware of the passage of time as endured. It has a sort of double consciousness of time, from without and from within. Hence he thinks that there must be something in the brain which acts as a timekeeper. The only sort of clock which could measure a directed-time would be one which indicated the degradation of energy to a lower or more unorganized level, *i.e.* an entropy clock ; for, as we saw above, ordinary clocks are neutral as between past and future. They only measure duration not direction of time. Whence he infers " that consciousness . . . may be guided by entropy-clocks in some portion of the brain. . . . And there is no reason why the generation of the random element (*i.e.* the amount of disorganization) in a special locality of the brain should not proceed fairly uniformly. In that case there will not be too great a divergence between the passage of time in consciousness and the length of the corresponding temporal relation in the physical world." The whole object of this argument is to demonstrate " that there is at least a one-to-one correspondence between the sequence of phases of the mind and a sequence of points in temporal relation."

This highly ingenious deduction, however, depends for its validity on overlooking several fundamental distinctions which we must bring to light. We saw, in an earlier chapter, that there is no evidence for the assumption that there is a one-to-one correspondence between mental and bodily events. The sole reason for the assumption is the implied dogma that we can only understand mental events by supposing them, in some way, to mirror physical events. But the two series of events belong to different orders of reality, and there is no reason to think that they ought to correspond ; or, at all events, those who think they ought to do so should provide reasons for this belief. There are, on the other hand, strong reasons to think that they cannot correspond. One thing may symbolically represent another without any point-to-point correspondence between the two. Where is the one-to-one correspondence between the flag of a country and the nation it represents ? If a mind may be said in some way to represent the particular brain with which it has connection there is no reason why it should have a one-to-one correspondence with it. Because a member of Parliament represents his constitutency he does not need to have a one-to-one correspondence with his constitutents. Let us consider, in this connection, the concept of organization, for this is an idea which has relevance both to body and to mind, since in some sense both are organized. Now disorganization was said above to be the only ground for believing in the real passage of time in the physical world. But in the psychical world the contrary holds, for the passage of time is an essential condition for bringing about such organization as we find amongst mental events. The difference between a mature and an immature mind is just this fact of organization. Here we see a fundamental disparity between the physical and the psychical ; the passage of time yielding disorganization in the one and organization in the other.

The concept of organization is in fact teleological and mental through and through. Thus, when the pieces are set out at the beginning of a game of chess they can only rightly be said to be organized if we have a game in view. Without the idea of the game there is nothing corresponding to organization and the pieces might be conceived as having been thrown down, at random, by one of those lucky chances which the calculus of probabilities assures us will occur if we go on throwing long enough. A malicious demon, ignorant of chess, might have done it to baffle our ideas. Suppose, however, the pieces are correctly set out and the game is played by two masters of chess. As it proceeds the arrangement of the pieces becomes more and more disorganized from the demon's or the scientific point of view ; and the amount of such disorganization varies roughly with the number of moves made or the time which has elapsed. But from the point of view of winning the game, *i.e.* from the mental standpoint, the pieces are becoming more and more organized; and the greater the amount of such organization the more chess-time has gone into the game. The idea of the game, or the purpose of chess-playing, entirely determines what shall be called organization or disorganization. At the beginning of an individual's experience all is, as James said, a big blooming buzzing confusion. Presentations come and go, but are not sorted out or organized into any coherent pattern. This is the work of mental activity or attention, and until the mind begins to deteriorate there is a continual growth and organization of experiences ; at all events in those whose minds are said to be cultivated. In the light of this, we should not expect to find any point-to-point correspondence in the two sets of sequences enumerated above.

But there are stronger grounds than this epistemological one for denying the correspondence, and these are purely psychological. The notion of time embedded in the space-time complex must somehow be derived from psychological experiences ; but this is not to say that it is identical with it. In fact the conceptual idea of time is obtained by rigorously excluding certain characteristics of perceptual time, *i.e.* time as endured, to which we must now devote some attention. All perception is tragic ; a sensation occurs and then is gone for ever, yielding the feeling of contrast expressed by ' now ' and ' then '. Conception is free from this fate, which is no doubt the reason that philosophers and scientists love to contemplate the world of ideas. But, to arrive at the notion of past and future as real items of our experience we must stick to the perceptual world, the world of impressions. It is the introduction of primitive memory and nascent expectation in our commerce with the material world that yields the experience of a ' now-past ' and a ' yet-to-come ' which are the very essence of our time experience. Without retentiveness and expectation of impressions there could be no experience of time. These, together with variations in the adjustment of attention to what is presented, are the ' material ' of time considered as a perceptual experience.

In order to render this clear let us have recourse to a simple symbolism in which A, B, C etc., represent impressions whilst a, b, c, etc., are their corresponding imaged representatives. It is to be remarked that such images need not be ' free ' in the sense of being capable of occurring apart from the actual impressions. In the early stages of experience all such images are ' tied ' to the corresponding percepts forming an integral and inseparable part of them. Thus, a young child seeing its milk bottle, in some primitive sense gets a foretaste of the milk, but there is no reason whatever to suppose that it can get an image of the taste apart from the sight of the bottle.

The bottle impression supports the taste image and is necessary to its arousal. Similarly, it is highly probable that all the images that lower animals have are implicated in the sense impressions; and are in no sense free. A dog's images, for example, are largely tied up in its smell impressions; so that a philosophical dog writing an account of the universe would be almost entirely limited to a scent terminology.

In order for the experience of time to emerge it is obviously necessary that the same series of impressions should recur; for a being limited to a single set of impressions could get no notion of time. Suppose the series of impressions A B C D E, in that order, to have occurred frequently in a person's experience. When on a future occasion A recurs the person's consciousness may be represented by A b c d e; such for instance would be the state of the child who perceives the preparations for his bottle of milk and expects to be fed. When he is just finishing his bottle his state of mind might be symbolized as a b c d E. The symbolism is not quite adequate, since the farther away from the impression that the image is, in the memory-train, the weaker it is; and the symbols do not represent this. At intermediate stages the state of mind may be represented by a B c d e, a b C d e and a b c D e. We may compare the experiences to a spot of light travelling across the series of impressions and lighting up each in its turn, leaving the extraneous members in lesser or greater depth of shadow according to the distance from the focus; just like a circle of light moving across the scale of a galvanometer. The illuminated member is the sense-impression, the greater or lesser shade the greater or less intensity of consciousness of the other members of the series. At the stage represented by a b C d e the first two members of the series are either after-sensations or primary-memory images sinking below the threshold of consciousness, *i.e.* their intensity is waning; whilst the last two, namely d and e, are images of expectation, or preperceptions, just arising above the threshold of consciousness, and their intensity is waxing. Such waxing and waning is due to the movements of attention by which we adjust ourselves to the coming

s

impressions or images. Thus, at the stage we are considering, attention is fully adjusted to the impression C which is in the focus of consciousness, and partially adjusted to d and e, whilst it is being relaxed as regards b and a ; all these latter four being in the margin of consciousness. These differences, which are comparable to distances in perspective, and which are *simultaneously perceived*, are the basis of our intuition or endurance of present, past and future. It is these differences of intensity in the contents of consciousness, combined with the forward looking aspect of attention, that give to our perception of time a sense or direction.

Now if we consider time as an element in the space-time concept this, as we have seen, has no direction or ' sense ' except in the one case of the second law of thermodynamics. The ot'.er characteristic of perceived time, namely a difference of intensity in its various parts, which distinguishes present from past and future has no corresponding feature in physical time. There are other characteristics, likewise, which distinguish the two. Chief amongst these is a character, which is common to all sensations, known by the name of protensity or felt endurance. No doubt there is something in the physical world corresponding to this endurance as felt, namely the duration of the stimulus. But, *as immediately experienced*, protensity or endurance varies from person to person, and also with the same person from time to time, depending on a personal *tempo*. As Shakespeare has it, " Time travels in divers paces with divers persons." In describing the Arabs of Southern Arabia Mr Bertram Thomas calls attention to their lack of the sense of time. " He has little sense of time, except as translated into distance ; he never learnt what an hour meant, even after days of experience, and as for minutes! they excited his mirth, making him wonder what strange finicky mortals we were to deal in such trifles." So that, whereas the objective stimulus may have the same duration, it by no means follows that the protensity is the same, for this is a purely subjective affair. Consequently the duration of the objective stimulus has no point-to-point correspondence with the *felt* protensity or endurance of the sensation. Such protensity is not felt so much as a duration but rather as a kind of intensity of the impression or experience.

For the sake of simplicity in explanation we have used symbols, and this apparently supports the one-to-one correspondence theory ; since each impression apparently leaves behind it a deposit of itself in the guise of an image. But this does violence to the psychological facts. When I listen to a melody, each note which is played no doubt has some effect on what I hear ; but what I hear is a gradually developing theme not a consecution of notes. When the melody is complete the impression is one whole, not a summation of parts. The earlier parts have faded away as impressions but are still present in the completed whole, for otherwise there would be no melody. Each consecutive impression has qualified the whole and made it a different whole ; an unsatisfying whole until all is complete. There is nothing in the state of consciousness at the end of the melody which corresponds to the fact that it was composed of a series of notes. In fact, an unmusical person may be totally unable to recall the series of chords and yet have a distinct melodious whole present to his mind.

It is a trite remark that presentations are revived in the order in which they have been attended to. Thus it is perfectly easy to repeat a poem we have learnt in the forward direction, but hopeless to attempt to repeat it backwards. The law of association has a forward direction or a sense. Hence it follows that the subjective residua of our acts of attention constitute ' temporal signs ' by which the times of our memory train are dated. Such temporal signs are entirely absent from the series of external events which gave rise to them, for the words of the poem are absolutely neutral as regards time. In other words we add to the successive presentations, as they come to us, time marks which are foreign to them. Without such temporal signs our memories instead of being a directed sequence would be chaotic. So that, here again, the one-to-one correspondence, which is assumed to hold between whatever physiological substratum is imagined for the separate impressions and the mental sequence, breaks down.

The notion of time as a co-ordinate in a space-time frame-work, which is the conceptual symbol which physics deals with has, therefore, very different characteristics from time as perceptually experienced. From the latter all differences of intensity or felt endurance and time-order are ruthlessly cut away in order to arrive at the former. Thus James Ward (5), to whose account of time perception I am greatly indebted, aptly summarizes the situation : " Our concrete time-experiences are due to the simultaneous representation of a series of definite presentations . . . the representations have certain marks or temporal signs due to acts or movements of attention, whereby the memory continuum is formed ; the rate of these movements or ' moments ' is approximately constant (depending on our *tempo*) ; and each moment itself is primarily experienced as part of a peculiar subjective intensity." This admirable summary of the perception of time, from the purely psychological standpoint, reveals to us the almost total disparity between the notion of time which is employed in natural science and the insight into time which is part of our every-day experience. It is hardly necessary after this account to consider where, in the brain, we must place our entropy clocks in order to account for time as a living experience. We can do without them ; as all our time experience rests on purely subjective factors with which the brain as a physical organ has no concern.

Exactly similar considerations apply to the perception of space. This has characteristics quite foreign to the geometry of space, which is constructed by eliminating all reference to the subjective standpoint. But when we are considering spatial perception the subjective factors are the all-important ones. There is a factor of extensity in all sensations which lies at the basis of our spatial perception ; but is not itself spatial, being a sort of intensity corresponding to the protensity of temporal perception previously considered. The region in which we should expect the point-to-point correspondence theory between mind and body to hold most perfectly is in the retina, for here there appears to be an arrangement of nerve fibres connected with the cortex well fitted to secure such correspondence. But the hope is a delusive one. For, an animal trained, for example, to discriminate patterns of white surfaces on a black background exercises the same discrimination when the black and white are interchanged. And he is equally unaffected if outlines are substituted for the corresponding surfaces, or even partial outlines which only suggest the original figure, provided that the same proportions are maintained. The stimuli which are psychologically equivalent to produce the discrimination involve different retinal elements to those which were actuated during the process of learning. Thus a habit may be formed by the activation of one set of receptors, and executed, unerringly, upon the stimulation of an entirely different set. The equivalence of stimuli for subjective activity is not therefore due to the excitation of common nervous elements.

Similarly, in man, where we can control the observations by securing introspective and linguistic evidence of what is happening instead of relying on inference, we find no convincing proof that there is a correspondence between the stimulation of definite retinal areas and sensory perception. The forms of scotoma do not correspond to the manifold shapes of the lesions. K. S. Lashley (6), for example, observed a " migraine scotoma in which the blind area retained a characteristic shape but drifted from the macula to the periphery of the visual field." The same is true of the retinal projection area in the brain. Even though this is in a fixed anatomical relationship to the retina " the functional organism plays over it just as the pattern of letters plays over the bank of lamps in an electric sign." A variable pattern of function shifts over a fixed anatomical pattern of elements. In the same way we have seen that the function of the various anatomical points in the ' motor cortex ' is variable, depending on temporal and other relations. The most that can be said has been said by Mr Lashley : " Definitely limited defects appear in the visual and tactile and to a lesser extent in the motor fields after limited lesions to the calcarine, postcentral and precentral gyri. In other sensory spheres and in all the more elaborate organization of behaviour, there is little evidence for an equal fineness of differentiation. The visual cortex represents the maximum of specialization of small units. In the somesthetic field there is also a cortical projection, but less finely differentiated. In other functions we find every degree of specialization up to the limit where all parts of the cortex participate equally in the same function."

Little can be said in favour of the one-to-one correspondence in the face of this summary of observed facts. The suspicion begins to arise that this dogma of correspondence, like many another, is due to the belief that ' function ' in the organic world is the same thing as function in the inorganic, because the term is the same. We must change our idea of ' function ' to suit the facts. Because the function of a machine depends on a one-to-one correspondence of the various parts in it and the movement as a whole, it does not in the least follow that the functions of the organism must be conceived after the same pattern. The theory of machine working is not the pattern for understanding the mind.

But if our terminology and ideas are faulty with regard to cortical functioning they are positively vicious when we consider nervous action in general. Here the mathematical bias is very obvious. Mathematicians require units to work with and can perform astonishing flights of reasoning when provided with them. Physical science, too, is dependent on sharply defined units. And physiologists have accordingly invented a unit for nervous action, the reflex. We saw, in an earlier chapter, that all modes of nervous activity from the spinal level upwards are conceived to be integrations of reflexes. The fundamental assumptions underlying this theory are that individual nervous arcs are specialized for particular functions, and that the synapses offer a definite resistance to the passage of nervous impulses. Habit, memory, instinct, heredity, etc., are all explained in terms of reflex arcs with varying resistances between the synapses. But there is no evidence for any specific function of the synapse, nor for varying resistances at different synapses, nor that this resistance is diminished by the passage of nervous impulses. All these assumptions are round about ways of expressing psychological facts in physiological terminology. As has been well pointed out, and the whole argument of this book substantiates it, " Psychology is to-day a more fundamental science than neuro-physiology. The latter offers few principles from which we can predict or define the normal organizations of behaviour, whereas the study of psychological processes furnishes a mass of factual material to which the laws of nervous action in behaviour must conform." Anybody who has read the preceding chapters can easily assure himself that this opinion is well grounded. The study of aphasia for example well bears out this view, for all the anatomical basis is suspect, and the facts have all been explained by Dr Henry Head and others in purely psychological terms. (7)

The reflex theory was invented to explain action on the spinal level, and is very successful, as a model, when restricted to such acts. One of the characteristics of a reflex response is its fatality; if a sufficiently strong stimulus is applied the action is inevitable. But there is nothing corresponding to this at the higher levels of action. Voluntary action is not inevitable or pre-determined by structure, and automatic actions do not depend on repeated stimuli. If physiologists had paid heed to Marshall Hall's careful use of the term reflex this unwarranted extension of the idea could not have occurred. An instructive instance of the extension of the reflex idea to regions where it does not apply is furnished by the so-called conditioned reflex. The only similarity between this and spinal reflexes is the name. Pavlov started out with definite intention of shewing that the mechanical view of nervous activity is the only justifiable view, and that no factors other than mechanical ones are at work. But we have seen that what he has really done is to provide a sound experimental basis for verifying the law of association. This law is mental from end to end, and could only be considered otherwise if experiments were restricted to animals and the mental factors merely inferred. Even so the explanation in physiological terms is hopelessly inadequate.

It is interesting to note that Dr A. Wohlgemuth (8), who performed experiments on memory and association, arrived at similar conclusions to mine on totally independent grounds. He was struck as I was by the similarity between certain conditions necessary to establish a conditioned reflex and those obtaining in forming an association of ideas. He thinks, however, that the associations between events at the cortical level is reversible whilst those at the lower physiological level of movements are irreversible. However that may be, there is no doubt at all that the kind of experiments that Pavlov has undertaken are only understandable in terms of mental functioning.

Conditioned reflex experiments performed on animals, however, tend to obscure the issue, since the interpretation is so much a matter of inference. No experiment, in fact, in which introspection is ruled out has any direct bearing on psychology and, therefore, on the mind-body problem. Fortunately, conditioned reflex experiments have been performed on human beings and these must be considered in detail. In one set of experiments the reflex studied was the knee jerk, actuated by a blow from a wooden hammer electrically controlled. (9) The conditioned stimulus was either a bell note, or a click in a pair of earphones, or a tactual stimulus obtained by letting a stylus fall on a finger. Out of 49 subjects who were tested, in groups of 9 or 10, conditioned patellar reflexes occured in 44. We shall describe the cases of those persons in which the conditioned responses were most effective. In these, the conditioned stimulus was the note of a bell which was sounded about one-third of a second before the blow on the knee was given. At irregular intervals during the course of the experiments the subjects were instructed, by printed directions, to clench the fists or say " ah " as soon as the bell rung. Thus, they might have to say " ah " at the fifth repetition of the bell, or clench the fist at the seventh, and so forth. To the rest of the conditioned stimuli they did not have to make any voluntary response. The remainder of the 49 persons had no such instructions.

It was found that the group of subjects who had to make the voluntary responses proved the most effective in establishing the conditioned reflex. The increased effectiveness was shewn by the smaller number of double stimuli (conditioned and unconditioned) needed to produce the conditioning, and by the increased extent of the knee jerk. The experimenter says that "when facilitation, in the form of a voluntary response to the conditioning stimulus, was used, conditioned knee jerks were obtained more than twice as frequently as when no facilitating reponse was used." Now what is the explanation of this curious and startling result ? If a physiological account of conditioned reflexes were possible these results would be incredible ; they simply could not occur. But if, as we suggested in an earlier chapter, a psychological explanation is the only sound one then the results are immediately intelligible. For, in psychological matters *attention* is a causal factor. And, without any bias one way or the other, the experimenter suggested as an explanation the preparation to give a voluntary response, such as clenching the fists, as soon as the conditioned stimulus occurs " directs the attention to the stimulus. This would probably give the stimulus a greater effectiveness, and therefore a better and more rapid conditioning might be expected." Here we see that, as in all other cases, where mind and body interact, the true causal factor is mental. Interesting evidence pointing to this conclusion has been obtained by investigations conducted by the National Fatigue Research Board into occupational neuroses. Telegraphist's and writer's cramp have long been regarded as neuro-muscular disturbances ; but it has been shewn that sufferers from these and similar complaints shew a high incidence of purely psychological disturbances.

An interesting confirmation of this view is presented by an investigation into what is known in psychology as ' perseveration.' By this term is meant the persistence of a sensory effect after the stimulus has ceased, or the spontaneous recurrence to consciousness of an experience without fresh stimulation, such as the running of a tune in a man's head. The first of these effects, if not the second, is due to a property of the nervous system, a sort of inertia which varies with different people. It may be measured by the rate at which a colour disc with green and red sectors must be rotated to produce the sensation of grey. With those in whom perseveration is strong the rate of rotation is less, for the one colour persists longer and so can be fused with the other at a lower number of revolutions. By an experimental investigation of this and other persisting effects Mr W. Lankes (10) tried to find out whether there was any correlation between this sort of perseveration and the qualities of persistence in character as estimated by observation of the persons examined. He failed to find any correlation between the perseverance qualities of behaviour and the phenomena of perseveration. Thence he concluded that " the absence of correlation between the two perseverances proves the independence of perseveration and will . . . and tends to shew that the self can modify, and directly counteract, its own nervous system and its innate tendency towards Perseveration or the opposite." If this investigation is sound, it shews that the mind is able to regulate the action of the body in defiance of the latter's physiological characteristics. Whether sound or not, this is the conclusion which our whole survey has suggested.

The fact of the matter is that the explanation of behaviour, even of purely organic behaviour, such as salivation, by means of conditioned reflexes is largely due to a loose use of terminology. It is assumed, without any justification, that the same mechanism is at work when a conditioned response is made as when behaviour depends on unconditioned stimuli. Hence the same name ' reflex action ' is applied to both. But there is nothing whatever to shew that action determined by a substituted stimulus has the same characteristics as native reactions ; and we have no business to call the former reflex action. For the appearance of the unconditioned response of salivation is determined by the strength of the stimulus, and increases as the latter increases. Whereas Messrs Winsor and Bayne (11) have shewn that for the conditioned reaction, on the other hand, a weak stimulus may be effective whilst a stronger stimulus invokes no response whatsoever. The unconditioned salivary response has all the character of a reflex activity and seems to be almost immune to fatigue.

Thus a twelve hour test of the glands shewed no evidence of diminution of secretion. But when we are dealing with the conditioned response the amount of secretion appears to depend on the state of hunger or satisfaction. " When the subject is in a state of complacency as far as food is concerned the conditioned salivary responses become very weak or disappear altogether." What is the sense, then, of calling the conditioned response a reflex action ?

As a result of our long analysis we may conclude that the bodily mechanism, in so far as it is not vegetative or automatic, is entirely responsive to mental factors. These are the controlling and regulating forces, and without them the nervous system is powerless. The supposition, that out of the combination of reflex activities higher activities emerge, has no factual evidence whatever, being simply an evasion of the problem of voluntary action. On the other hand there are numerous examples within our experience of the degradation of voluntary activities into semi-automatic acts. Every time we cultivate a bodily habit we get an instance of this ; not, indeed, of the production out of a voluntary act of a reflex act, for the latter is a pure abstraction ; but of the becoming non-volitional or semi-volitional of what was once done with full consciousness. The theory of lapsed conscious striving is founded on observed fact, whereas the theory of the development of conscious acts out of reflex acts is a pure myth ; emergent evolution notwithstanding.

Let us, however, leave the reflex arc on one side and consider the doctrine of emergent evolution in general as presented in the masterly treatise of that name by Mr Lloyd Morgan (12), as this is largely concerned with the relation of body to mind. According to this doctrine, at some stage of the history of the world, life emerged from the inorganic world, and at a later stage consciousness emerged. Neither life nor consciousness was in any way involved in the lower forms from which they emerged, but these new relations came into existence as such novel facts that no conceivable logical analysis could have detected their possibility at prior stages ; they just happened. Conscious processes emerged from physiological processes when these latter reached a certain stage of complexity. "What emerges at any given level affords an instance of a new kind of relatedness of which there are no instances at lower levels. The world has been successively enriched through the advent of vital and conscious relations. This we must accept with ' natural piety ', as Mr Alexander puts it. If it be found as somehow given, it is to be taken just as we find it. . . . In a physical system wherein life has emerged, the way things happen is raised to a higher plane. In an organism within which consciousness is emergent a new course of events depends on its presence. In a person in whom reflective thought is emergent behaviour is sustained at a higher level. . . . Strike out all guiding consciousness and behaviour is that appropriate to the level of life. Strike out life and the course of events drops down to the physical level. The new relations emergent at each higher level guide and sustain the course of events distinctive of that level."

After this clear presentation of the doctrine Mr Lloyd Morgan goes on to consider the order in which mental qualities arise, and classifies them as sensory data, perceptions, and contemplative thought, in ascending order of emergence. Each is supposed to have emerged at a later historical stage ; and each, presumably, was not foreseeable at a prior stage of evolution.

As a philosophical doctrine I am perfectly willing to accept this, if not with natural piety at least with natural diffidence due to such eminent authority. It is possible that evolution as a whole becomes more intelligible when viewed from this standpoint ; and creative evolution is certainly the only kind of evolution which *is* intelligible. But from the psychological standpoint the theory is hard to justify. Sensory data may be the most elementary of the constitutents of consciousness as revealed by analysis, but that is no reason to assume that they are prior in time to perceptions or thought. Such data are the highly elaborated abstractions of philosophers, not the units that the mind works with. They are obtained by a double dose of abstraction ; first the subject perceiving them is torn away from the context, and secondly the rest of the universe of which they are a part. What the first experiences of a living being are like, nobody knows or can know, but we may be quite sure that they are not like sense-data. If we may make a guess they are more akin to feelings.

But we know what thought is like. And there is nothing, within our experience, to lead us to think that it is evolved out of sense perceptions. What our experience teaches us is that states of full consciousness give rise to events in which consciousness is at a minimum. We learn, with great effort, to perform a task and, on repetition, this becomes easier so that attention is less necessary. Finally the task becomes quasi-automatic. All our intellectual habits are instances of this. So that the course of evolution, as far as our direct experience gives us any insight into it, is not in the least like what the philosophical view would have us believe. Voluntary action, accompanied by reflective thought, gives way to subconscious action in which thought is at a minimum. If we like to carry speculation further we may surmise that the fully conscious becomes more and more unconscious. This is what the psychological facts lead us to ; not to the development of consciousness out of the unconscious, but of the unconscious out of the conscious. It was on grounds somewhat similar to these that Samuel Butler (13) attempted to explain the course of evolution, and though his view was speculative, it stuck to the facts ; and from the psychological standpoint it was unexceptionable. Physiological action, in brief, emerges out of psychological, and instead of so-called reflex action being the unit out of which higher action is developed, the kind of action which it suggests has arisen out of conscious activities. I am not at all certain that Mr Lloyd Morgan would wholly dissent from this view when he is speaking as a psychologist and not as a philosopher. For, as a philosopher, he is very careful, before he traces the emergence of life from matter, and mind from life, to explain that the substratum of the universe has two ultimate aspects, psychical and physical. So that the world for him, like for Spinoza, is both psychical and physical. What emerges at the stage of mind is not the psychical from the non-psychical ; but particular qualities of the psychical, or new relations, which did not occur before. I am not sure that this is the correct interpretation, but it is undoubtedly intelligible to consider mind as emerging from something that is psychical, and unintelligible to regard it as emerging from a body that is purely material.

It has become very evident by now that the mind-body relation has been obscured by a large number of unfounded assumptions derived from the epistemology and ontology of an earlier age, and the obscurities of the science of neurology. Before I give my own solution, which I hope does not involve equally ungrounded assumptions, it is desirable to consider one further view which has sufficient truth in it to be misleading. This is the belief that we only know the minds of others by an indirect inference from the sense-data which their bodies yield to us. Such a view leads logically to solipsism, or the theory that the only mind of which I have any direct experience, and therefore which I know certainly to exist is my own ; and all other minds are inferences from their bodies. The behaviourists, as I interpret them, go one step further and deny that my own mind exists ; that too being known to me only through my bodily behaviour. The clearest statement of the inferential nature of our knowledge of other minds that I am familiar with was that given by Professor E. P. Bowne. (14)

" No thoughts leave the mind of one and cross into the mind of the other. When we speak of an exchange of thought even the crudest mind knows that this is a mere figure of speech. To perceive another's thought, we must construct his thought within ourselves. This thought is our own and is strictly original with us. At the same time we owe it to the other ; and if it had not originated with him, it would probably not have originated with us. But what has the other done ? This : by an entirely mysterious world-order, the speaker is enabled to produce a series of signs which are totally unlike the thought, but which, by virtue of the same mysterious order, act as a series of incitements upon the hearer, so that he constructs within himself the corresponding mental state. The act of the speaker consists in availing himself of the proper incitements. The act of the hearer is immediately only the reaction of the soul against the incitement. All communion between finite minds is of this sort."

Now I am not concerned to deny that this is a correct view of the nature of external perception. It may well be that our sensations are to us merely symbols of the existence of an external world. For in no true sense of the word do we perceive sensations. Sensations are lived through or endured and are the signs by which we perceive the external world. The sensation has a thought-reference to some object, and it is this object which I perceive, not the sensation. Sensations direct me to objects but are not themselves objects for me. They are, if you like, the media through which objects are perceived. Just as in looking through a pair of perfectly clean blue spectacles I perceive a world of blue objects, but not the glasses, so by virtue of my sensations I perceive other things than themselves. My sensations, as experiences, are diaphanous to me just as clean glasses are. If somebody, whilst I am asleep, substitutes a pair of red spectacles and I am completely ignorant of the change that has been made, I shall, on awaking, perceive red objects around me. A change in my sensory experiences, therefore, produces a corresponding change in my perceptions without the necessity of my being immediately aware of the sensations. It is possible that to a more primitive consciousness sensations themselves may be items in awareness, and that mental evolution consists in passing beyond this stage to a stage of thought-reference. This, if I understand it, is the doctrine of emergent evolution. The reason which prompts me to accept this view is that our most primitive sensations are our organic sensations. It is because such sensations are perceived directly that their thought-reference is so vague and uncertain. My organic sensations tell me nothing worth knowing about my body. It takes a skilled physician to interpret the meaning of my organic sensations and to say to what they refer. Left to myself I can only describe them vaguely and I even locate them erroneously. In the case of painful sensations the thought-reference is somewhat more definite but the pain, in so far as it is painful, baffles any thought-reference at all, as we experience in the case of violent toothache.

But whereas sensations, though immediately endured, are not perceived, but the objects to which they refer, the same is not true of other minds. It is no doubt true, that if we disregard telepathy, we can only get into touch with another mind by way of his body. But this, in no sense, implies that the contact, when we do make it, is an inference or is indirect. If we could not get into communion directly with other minds we could never get into touch at all. The matter may be made clear by considering another branch of knowledge. John Locke attempted to prove that there were no innate logical principles in the mind, on the ground that new born children and primitive men were unaware of such principles. He argued that, if they were innate, we must be born with them, which, of course, is strictly true but quite irrelevant. Though such logical principles, which form the foundation of reasoning, are innate it requires the stimulus of experience to make us aware of their significance. We have, as it were, to learn the language in which these principles are expressed before we become aware that we possess these principles within our consciousness. But the fact, that we only become aware of them as the result of experience, does not imply that they are inferences from experience, as the sensationalist philosophers so long maintained. The experience by which we are made aware of them is inadequate to establish them, though it is essential to our awareness.

In a similar fashion the knowledge of minds other than one's own is innate, and as soon as the child has had sufficient experience he realizes that this must be so. He, moreover, realizes it at an age when it is utterly inconceivable that any process of construction or indirect inference leading to such a conclusion is possible. It takes a philosophic mind, by a roundabout course of reasoning, to throw any doubt on this direct knowledge of others' minds. And, no doubt, this epistemological theory is valuable as an exercise in philosophy, but it has nothing whatever to do with our direct psychological awareness of the fact that other people perceive and feel as we do. I do not perceive a machine, as Descartes thought, when I perceive another body similar to my own ; but a thinking body. For this reason I am in entire agreement with Professor Whitehead (15), who on the philosophical basis of considering all bodies as organisms arrives at the same conclusion. " A body for an external observer is the aggregate of the aspects for him of the body as a whole, and also of the body as a sum of parts. For the external observer the aspects of shape and of sense-objects are dominant, at least for cognition. But we must also allow for the possibility that we can detect in ourselves direct aspects of the mentalities of higher organisms. The claim that the cognition of alien mentalities must necessarily be by means of indirect inferences from aspects of shape and of sense-objects is wholly unwarranted by this philosophy of organism." This seems to me so true and obvious that I can only assume that those who hold a different view must be obsessed by the idea that we know matter more intimately than we can ever know mind.

But as we have so repeatedly insisted, and must urge again, our knowledge of mind is direct insight ; both of our own and of other minds. Of our own it is so patent that not even a philosopher has ever doubted it. It is from the mental side, therefore, that any enlightenment on the mind-body problem must be sought. For here alone are we in direct touch with a reality which we cannot doubt. Our direct knowledge of the external world is merely a symbolic knowledge and any knowledge of reality outside us, except mental reality, is an indirect or inferential knowledge. Some, indeed, like Mr Bertrand Russell, have gone so far as to assert that there is nothing at all behind the symbols, or that the sum total of all appearances constitutes the external world. If we include among the appearances the possible as well as the actual appearances, a good case can apparently be made out for this strange belief. If ten men look at an object there are ten different appearances ; and we can imagine an infinite number of observers to collect all the other possible appearances. This collection of appearances might then, in a logical sense, be interpreted to constitute the existence of the object. I am far from saying that this is

T

a tenable view, but it is a possible one and might serve, for aught I know, all the purposes of physics. But for the existence of a mind this view is not even a possible one.

Suppose an infinite collection of Boswells all to have produced lives of Dr Johnson, each from his own point of view. Would this be a complete account of the life of the lexicographer? Obviously not; for the most important point of view is left out of account, the point of view of the man himself. This is the only angle from which an inside view is possible, the only subjective standpoint in the whole collection. The peculiarly privileged position of this standpoint gives a direct insight into the nature of Being obtainable in no other way. What this reveals is reality; and anything else which has a claim to the same name, must occupy a similar point of view. To understand the nature of the reality of an electron we should have to occupy the point of view of an electron. The biographies of the electron from the physicist's point of view are written from outside positions. It is for this reason that I am in sympathy with those who maintain, with Spinoza, that everything in the universe must be considered from a psychical as well as from a physical standpoint, that is from the inside as well as the outside aspect.

Having hacked our way through a forest of misconceptions we can now hope to tackle the mind-body relation. The real difficulty that faces us lies in the fact that this relation is unique and consequently there is nothing to compare it with. Hence, for any further elucidation we are reduced to analogies, and these always carry misleading implications. Let us see what light can be derived from such analogies. The mind-body relation may be compared to that of a learned society to its members. Each member or group of members is an organ carrying out part of the purposes of the society; and the society exists as long as these purposes are being pursued. Now the only way of explaining the nature of the society is to understand the purposes which the organization is striving to accomplish. Any other view than this is subsidiary, external or irrelevant. We must take our standpoint within the society or we shall misconceive it. The existence of any particular member is quite immaterial since the society exists so long as it is carrying out its purposes.

Or we may compare the mind-body relation to that which subsists between the composition of a work of art, such as a lyric, and the material out of which it is apparently constructed, namely language. It will be seen, at once, that it would be ridiculous to expect any light to be thrown on the poetry by an examination of the words considered apart from the poem ; as for instance when found in a dictionary. Nevertheless this was the blunder made for a long time by schoolmasters who imagined they were cultivating an appreciation of Shakespeare by digging out the etymology of his words. There obviously is a relation between the words and the poetry, but it is only perceived by getting inside the lyric from the appreciative standpoint. So the mind-body displays activities which cannot be discerned except from the standpoint of subjectivity. And we have had abundant opportunities to realize that whenever the attempt has been made to describe the relation by using physical or physiological concepts it has always broken down. Why, indeed, should we expect such concepts to be applicable, except on the view that the relation is not unique ? In an earlier chapter we examined the notion of mental energy but found that this was unintelligible if the concept had its physical significance. And, again, we investigated the notion of mental activity, and decided that it was not intelligible unless we referred to a realm in which principles and ideals were the determining concepts ; a spiritual realm.

Thus we are led to the view that when our concepts are derived from the spiritual sphere of activity an explanation of the relation is possible ; not otherwise. For, if we start without any physical preconceptions, it is feasible to discern how the mind-body carries out the spiritual purposes of the person. There are, in fact, four terms to the relation we are investigating ; namely the person or ego, spiritual forces, the mind and the living body. And it is by ignoring the first two of these that the irreconcilable contradictions, we so often encountered in our quest, are due.

To revert to our analogy ; a poem cannot be considered in terms of concepts derived from the study of words, nor in terms of its form apart from the words. What we need, in addition, are terms derived from the system of æsthetic values. Only this latter system throws any light on the inspiration of the poem ; since it is the inspiration alone which converts such unpromising material as dead words and bare forms into the spiritual reality of poetry. Mathematicians have often amused themselves with the thought that by taking all the words in a language and sorting them, at random, for an infinite time we should, by the laws of probability, get every poem that has ever, or can ever, be written. If this is considered as more than an idle play on the meaning of the word infinite, then it might be possible to say that the sorting of words determined the composition of the poem. This would be analogous to the consideration of the mind-body problem in terms of two factors. But those who do not delight in mathematical puzzles, and who do not believe that poetry, not even modern poetry, can be written by sorting out the words in a dictionary, even a rhyming dictionary, naturally search for the poet in order to account for the origin of verse ; and he corresponds to the third factor in the situation. A poet without genius or inspiration cannot produce real poetry and the source of such inspiration provides us with the fourth term in the relation. Physiological psychologists can do without three of these terms and give a complete explanation of the composition of the poem by means of brain cells and fibres alone. Philosophers require only two sets of terms, sense-data and the laws of probability and they, too, can adequately explain the origin of the poetry to their own satisfaction. The man untutored in these profundities goes on demanding the poet and his inspiration and is unsatisfied without them ; for he thinks that these alone give a satisfying explanation of the composition of the lyric. Leave out these two and the whole remains an inexplicable mystery.

The mind-body problem thus splits evidently into two separate parts, namely, that the living body is directed by mental factors, whilst the mind is controlled by spiritual forces.

The former of these considerations has been so abundantly dealt with in the preceding chapters that nothing more need be added. We pass to the second.

Many of the perplexities considered in the previous chapter arise from a confusion between two uses of the term mind. The mind that is contemplated when we are dealing with physiological psychology is not the same thing as the mind conceived as a subject or ego. Mind is used in two different senses ; as what has been called ' psychoplasm ' which is associated with and supplies the directing forces of the bioplasm, and which together with it constitutes a unity ; and as ego or subject for whom the unified psycho-bioplasm is an instrument for carrying out his purposes. When a sensation, for example, arises as the result of stimulating a nerve, this constitutes a modification or change in the psychoplasm. But some subject or ego is aware of this change. The sensation is owned ; it does not float about in the world at large, but belongs to some ego. This fact is so necessary that if we attempt to ignore it we are driven to the absurdity of supposing that each separate sensation has its own soul or ego which knows it. For known a sensation must be. Much misapplied ingenuity has been displayed by many psychologists and some philosophers in building up the structure of our knowledge on the basis of material, none of which is known to anybody. If, however, we recognize the ego or subject as an essential constituent in all knowledge or human activity, the problem that confronts us is the relation of this subject to the organic whole composed of mind and body. And the only concepts in terms of which this relationship is describable are spiritual ones, in which all the terms are terms expressing values.

Mr W. E. Johnson, whose interest in psychology was confined to its purely formal aspect as embodied in its logic, adopted a point of view which, in one respect, is so close to mine that I cannot refrain from a long quotation. (16) " The judgment which distinguishes the higher human volitions attributes *value* to possible existents, and in certain relevant cases comparative values to different alternatives ; such judgments predicating of their objects characters which are intrinsic to them, in the sense that they are entirely independent of the likes and dislikes of the person judging. . . . When objects are characterized by such adjectives as good or beautiful, they can properly be said to be raised into a realm of reality removed from that realm in which reference is made merely to predicates based upon qualities of sensation, or upon the scientifically developed properties of continuants. At any rate these adjectives ' good ' and ' beautiful ' are imposed upon their objects *in an act which is quite other than the analytico-descriptive* characteristics made by what we call science. . . . With regard to the influence of such judgments upon Conation, it may be that an attitude is necessarily evoked which tends to stimulate the thinker to produce so far as possible the kind of object to which value is attached in his judgment. If so, *a judgment of value of this kind may be said to be by itself the sufficient cause of a direct act of will* " (later italics all mine).

It is thus evident that, in order to account for an act of volition, logic is powerless unless it calls in the aid of spiritual forces. Strange indeed would it be if psychologists could dispense with them. The neglect of them may, perhaps, account for some of their perplexities in handling the mind-body problem. In any case it is illuminating to observe that the most acute of formal logicians declared the bankruptcy of scientific logic to cope with the question of the will ; and that he thought that spiritual concepts, by themselves, could be motive forces where acts of human volition were concerned. I am quite sure he was right ; and his refutation of the dependence of subjective activity on neurology, to which I called attention in an earlier chapter, shews that he had gone some way towards disentangling the four factors which are essential to understanding the mind-body relation.

These considerations enable us to deal with the question of the freedom of the will which has vexed theologians and philosophers for so long. Psychologists have also taken up the problem, but the only contribution they have made to it is to define freedom in a peculiar way. Freedom means, for them, self-determination, *i.e.* a man is free in so far as his thoughts and actions are determined by his self. In other words they are strictly calculable from a complete knowledge of the self and its present circumstances. This seems to me to imply that freedom and determinism are the very same thing ; or that one particular form of determinism guarantees the freedom of the will. I am not sure whether the self contemplated in this view means the self as subject or the self as psychoplasm attached to a particular body. If it means the latter, and if this is combined with the belief that every mental event must have a bodily accompaniment, then it is hard to see how anything can be said in its favour.

Why is it considered necessary to preserve calculability or predictability in discussing this problem ? For that is what self-determinism implies. The reason, no doubt, is that it has been long supposed that the only scientific way of studying mind is to use the concepts of natural science. As, until recently, determinism was supposed to be absolutely necessary to science, and indeterminism quite inconceivable, psychologists thought that they were bound to square their doctrines with the principles of determinism. Hence they combined the doctrine of freedom (which is the antithesis of determinism) with the concept of determinism and produced the hybrid self-determination. No doubt, also, they feared that any other view would lay them open to the charge of believing in purely capricious action. The eagerness with which politicians have seized on the notion of self-determination as an equivalent for freedom ought to have warned us that the idea was suspicious.

But determinism is a dogma of an epistemology which is no longer held by modern physics, and we can therefore preserve our reputation as scientists by discarding it in psychology. Professor G. P. Thomson, in his interesting study of the atom, thus neatly sums up the situation (17) : " From the philosophical point of view the most important feature of the recent quantum mechanics is its strong trend away from determinism. Since the time of Newton, it had been taken almost for granted that, at least in dead matter, every particle moved in obedience to exact and definite laws. It was supposed that if the initial position and velocity of every particle of a group free from outside influence were known exactly, and if the proper laws had been found, it would be possible to calculate the position of each particle at any later time. The whole behaviour of the system was determinate. . . . The theoretical possibility was believed to be a real truth, and it obliged those who wished to believe in the free will of human beings to suppose some profoundly fundamental difference between the behaviour of the atoms in a man's brain or nerves, from that of the same atoms forming part of dead matter.

" The newer view makes this unnecessary. Most of the laws of atomic physics are expressed as probabilities, which, of course, become certainties when a sufficient number of independent events are concerned to make statistics apply . . . there is an inherent uncertainty or power of choice in the world, but with this proviso, that the power of choice is exercised in such a way that in the bulk average laws are obeyed. Certain events are regarded as ' equally probable ' choices of nature. There is thus no physical argument against free will whatever may be the metaphysical objections."

It was previously stated that many of our baffling difficulties in psychology rose from the taking over of the logic of the physical sciences into the realm of mind. But physics, as we see, readily abandons its own epistemology to fit the new facts of observation. Whereas we, as psychologists, always follow in their wake and feel that we must conform to them even when we are dealing with relationships unknown to natural science. But there is no reason whatever why this should be our attitude. And in any case self-determination is an attempt to get the worst out of both possible worlds ; to preserve determinism which is no longer valid in the physical realm, and to equate it with freedom   There is no purpose served by trying to make psychological concepts fit into a physical scheme ; and our previous examination of the characteristics of temporal perception has justified this scepticism.

Kant (18) knew better than this, though he believed in the doctrine of universal determinism in the realm of science ; and there was no reason, in his day, why he should not. But he rescued the doctrine of the freedom of the will by calling in the noumenal world to redress the balance of the world of science. " Every rational being," he says, " reckons himself *qua* intelligence as belonging to the world of understanding, and it is simply as an efficient cause belonging to that world that he calls his causality a *will.* On the other hand he is also conscious of himself as a part of the world of sense in which his actions which are mere appearances [phenomena] of that causality are displayed . . . but these actions as belonging to the sensible world must be viewed as determined by other phenomena, namely, desires and inclinations. . . . Since, however, *the world of understanding contains the foundation of the world of sense, and consequently of its laws also,* and accordingly gives the law to my will (which belongs wholly to the world of understanding) directly, it follows that, although on the one side I must regard myself as a being belonging to the world of sense, yet on the other side I must recognize myself as subject as an intelligence to the law of the world of understanding, *i.e.* to reason, which contains this law in the idea of freedom."

Those who still hanker after the epistemology of the physical sciences have, however, in the present age another obstacle to encounter, namely the doctrine of emergence. According to this doctrine perfectly new properties may emerge at any stage of evolution and these must be accepted without any hope of further explanation. If such realities as life, consciousness, etc., have emerged it would indeed be a tragicomedy played by nature if freedom could not emerge ; especially as it no longer has to fear the ghost of determinism. Freedom implies the possibility of making a decision on grounds which previously have made no appeal to the self. This, I take it, is the meaning of conversion in religion. A man makes a decision entirely opposed to his whole past self ; which may be loosely expressed as the emergence of a new self. But this would be impossible if freedom meant self-determination. When we are considering the problem at higher levels of human activity (and such consideration alone gives the problem any significance) a new set of concepts has to be taken into account. At such levels the possibility of freedom is concerned with the power of choosing between alternatives on the grounds of *value* instead of being influenced merely by desire. And values are discerned or appreciated, but not created by the subject who evaluates. The appreciation of values, and the development of a self to whom they have some appeal, is the ultimate ground for believing in the freedom of the will. Such discernment creates new motives of activity ; and we saw above that the logic of the natural sciences provides no explanation of this, but has to accept it as a brute fact. It was, no doubt, with some such idea at the back of his mind that Kant founded the freedom of the will on a transcendental self. But this was mainly a metaphysical dodge to allow him to retain the doctrine of determinism in the natural world. And this is no longer necessary.

We saw, earlier in the chapter, that the distinction between appearance and reality only forces itself on our attention if we confine our view to the world of physical objects. But with regard to one's own consciousness we are able to take an inside view, by living through it. So that the distinction between appearance and reality has no significance where the ego is concerned ; to live is to be. The mind, as subject, endowed with self-consciousness is on a different plane of reality owing to the possibility of taking this subjective standpoint. Such a view point gives us observations and knowledge obtainable in no other way. We have, therefore, a realization of freedom which is direct and requires no external backing. The guarantee of its possibility is obtained by living through it and experiencing it. Everybody who has experienced the difference between obeying an order from a superior and acting on his own initiative knows perfectly well what freedom *feels like*. Any outside observer who thinks this freedom an illusion must be prepared to explain why the illusion arises only in the latter case, for the consciousness of this freedom undoubtedly exists. In his very able book *The Psychology of Intelligence and Will* Mr H. G. Wyatt (19) maintains, and I agree with him, that the characteristic of volition is not conation but initiative. All talk about balancing

or weighing motives and other physical analogies is pure
moonshine. The extent to which our actions are determined
by our intelligence is the extent to which freedom is assured
and felt. " Volition at its highest level is the creation of
motive. On no other basis can we admit it. For once we
grant that all human activity is either instinctively impelled
or impelled by habits derived from instincts, the volitional
consciousness becomes meaningless. It is an illusion, and has
no place in human behaviour at all. Initiation ceases to be
initiation as soon as it is resolved into original impulse, for
our original impulses are given us : they entail not initiation,
but its opposite."

The freedom of the will, which is directly experienced, is
all the justification we require for believing in it ; unless we
are committed to views which it is the whole purpose of this
book to reject. A psychology which ignores the vital difference
between experience, as experienced, and experience as viewed
by an outside observer misses the whole significance of conscious
life. And it is only outside observers trying to construct
epistemologies which shall measure physical objects and
mental events with the same yard stick who have ever thought
of doubting the validity of this direct experience of freedom.
Moreover, what in the name of all that is psychological is " the
will " ? We might as well talk of " the headache." There is
no such thing as a headache ; there are only persons suffering
from headaches. Physicians have long abandoned this mode
of talking and consider not the headache but the patient.
Let us follow suit and no longer think of the freedom of the
will but the freedom of the subject or person. If we do this
we see that will divorced from intelligence is an empty
abstraction. A man is free when and so far as he acts in
accordance with principles or ideals or makes use of his
intelligence. For it is the distinguishing mark of intellect to
go beyond the sense-given and distinguish general truths and
ultimate values. Thus, in so far as spiritual values appeal
to a man, so far is he free.

We may end this volume with a suggestion, which our
treatment has led to but which will require a further volume

to develop, concerning the immortality of the soul. The ancient Egyptians, in spite of their belief in the transmigration of the soul, were so convinced that the body was in some way necessary to its preservation that, when they could, they spent large sums in embalming the body. And this belief, that mortality is bound up with the dissolution of the body has, at all times, rendered the conception of immortality difficult. Now if the mind is a function of the brain it is hard to see where the Egyptians were wrong. But we have learnt that this view rests on a confusion between two different uses of the term mind ; the mind as psychoplasm and the mind as ego, soul or subject. Most of the discussions concerning the relation of mind to body have asumed only the former meaning of mind. It is so obvious, as hardly to be worth pointing out, that a sensation must be originated by some bodily mechanism. When the body dies there is consequently no possibility of a sensation arising. Now this has always carried with it the implication that mental imagery is subject to the same limitation, and the still more unjustified assumption that ideas are dependent on the body in the same way that sensations are.

The edge of this objection has been turned in the chapter on mental imagery, where it was shewn that such images are entirely subjective, dependent that is to say solely on the subject or ego. Their arousal has, of course, presupposed the occurrence of sensations ; but their existence in no way demands the continued existence of sensations. The contrary view presupposes that they are copies of sensation, and this we have seen to be a soulless blunder. All our subjective acts are dependent for their first arousal on some presentation, but none of them assumes the continued existence of such objects. Presentations are modifications of the psychoplasm not of the soul. No doubt such modifications lead to changes in the soul's activity but that is no reason for confusing the former with the latter.

In the last resort the question of the immortality of the soul can only be discussed in terms of concepts derived from religion. But what I am concerned to maintain is that the psychological objections against the belief, on the grounds of the mind-body relation, are due to faulty reasoning. If the view I have put forward is well founded, when a man contemplates the world of values the permanent effects on him are purely subjective. His being is steeped and dyed in what he experiences ; so that nobility of soul arises from the pursuit of what is of permanent worth. And it is the destiny of man to foster such commerce with ultimate values in the confident hope that what is so acquired, as it does not depend on the body, can never pass away.

REFERENCES

CHAPTER I.—PSYCHOLOGICAL PHYSIOLOGY.

1. DESCARTES. *De l'homme.* Paris, 1664.
2. J. P. MAHAFFY. *Descartes.* Blackwood, 1902, from which the translation is taken. Or see the last paragraph in *L'homme* of which this is a translation.
3. A. S. EDDINGTON. *Nature of the Physical World,* p. 209. Cambridge Univ. Press, 1928.
4. EDINGER UND FISCHER. Ein Mensch ohne Grosshirn. *Archiv. f. d. ges. Physiologie,* 1913.
5. G. ELLIOT SMITH. *Evolution of Man,* Ch. I. Oxford University Press, 1924.
6. H. PIÉRON. *Thought and the Brain,* Ch. I. Int. Lib. Psych. Kegan Paul, 1927.
7. H. HEAD. *Aphasia and Kindred Disorders,* Pt. IV, Ch. 1. Cambridge University Press, 1926.
8. W. JAMES. *Principles of Psychology,* Vol. I, Ch. 2. Macmillan.
   This chapter gives Meynert's scheme and his diagram. The diagram has been widely copied and assumed to be founded on physiological research. Whereas it is pure psychology rendered pictorially, as most other diagrams are.
9. C. S. SHERRINGTON. *Integrative Action of the Nervous System.* Constable, 1911.
   Essential for the study of reflex action.

CHAPTER II.—PSYCHOLOGICAL PHYSIOLOGY.

1. G. F. STOUT. *Manual of Psychology,* 4th ed., Bk. I, Ch. 2. W. B. Clive.
2. E. D. ADRIAN. *The basis of sensation.* Christophers, 1928.
   This should be read by all students of psychology, being packed tight with sound observations.
3. L. LAPICQUE. Principe pour une theorie du fonctionnement nerveux. *Revue Générale des Sciences,* Vol. 21, 1910.
4. J. P. PAVLOV. *Conditioned Reflexes,* translated by Anrep. Oxford University Press, 1927.
5. HALDANE. *Mechanism, Life and Personality.* Murray, 1921.
6. L. L. THURSTONE. *The Nature of Intelligence.* Int. Lib. Psych. Kegan Paul, 1924.
7. E. R. GUTHRIE. Conditioning as a principle of learning. *Psychol. Review,* Vol. 37, 1930.
8. J. P. PAVLOV. *Op. cit.,* Ch. 15.
9. J. P. PAVLOV. *Op. cit.,* Chs. 17 and 18.

CHAPTER III.—PHYSIOLOGICAL PSYCHOLOGY.

1. H. C. WARREN. *History of Association Psychology.* Constable, 1921.
   This gives Hartley's views at length. In order to appreciate them fully it is desirable to consult his *Observations on Man.*

2. M. FOSTER. *Lectures on history of Physiology,* Ch. 10. Camb. Univ. Press, 1901.

3. W. JAMES. *Text Book of Psychology,* Chs. 16, 18, 19.
   James copied most of his views on this and kindred matters from Hartley and acknowledged his debt. Others have copied them without acknowledgment.

4. J. B. WATSON. *Psychology from the standpoint of a behaviourist,* Ch. 8. Lippincott.

5. C. FOX. *Educational Psychology,* Ch. 5. Int. Lib. Psych. Kegan Paul.
   I have shewn in this book that the whole notion of unvarying pathways in the nervous system is invalid.

6. FRANZ AND LASHLEY. Retention of habits, etc. *Psychobiology.* Camb. Univ. Press, Vol. 1, 1917.

7. FRANZ AND LASHLEY. Effects of cerebral destruction, etc. *Psychobiology,* Vol. 1, 1917.
   These papers and the method employed are fundamental.

8. K. S. LASHLEY. *Brain Mechanisms and Intelligence.* University of Chicago Press, 1929.
   Everybody who wishes to understand cortical functioning must read this.

9. K. S. LASHLEY. *Op. cit.,* Ch. 3.

10. K. S. LASHLEY. *Op. cit.,* Ch. 10.

11. W. E. JOHNSON. *Logic,* Pt. 3, Ch. 8. Camb. Univ. Press, 1924.

12. C. D. BROAD. *Mind and its place in Nature,* Ch. 3. Int. Lib. Psych. Kegan Paul, 1925.

13. OGDEN AND FRANZ. On cerebral motor control, etc. *Psychobiology.* Camb. Univ. Press, 1917.

14. K. S. LASHLEY. (1) Studies in cerebral functions. *Psychobiology,* Vol. 2, 1918 ; (2) *Journal of Comparative Psychology.* Baltimore, Vol. 1.

15. *Brain Mechanisms, etc.,* Ch. 8.

16. MARSHALL HALL. On the reflex functions of the medulla oblongata, etc. *Phil. Transac. of Royal Society.* London, 1833.

17. MARSHALL HALL. Memoirs of the Nervous System. London, 1837. New Memoirs on the nervous system. London, 1843. Synopsis of the diastaltic nervous system. London (undated).
   These four articles are well worthy of close reading. They contain much historical information and are written in a broad scientific spirit. The observations are admirable.

18. K. S. LASHLEY AND J. BALL. Spinal Conduction and Kinæsthetic Sensitivity, etc. *Journ. of Comparative Psychol.,* Vol. 9, 1929.

CHAPTER IV.—PHYSIOLOGICAL PSYCHOLOGY.

1. H. HEAD. *Aphasia and Kindred disorders of Speech.* Camb. Univ. Press, 1926.
One of the best treatises on the mind-body problem. See especially Pt. 4, Ch. 4.

2. S. A. KINNEIR WILSON. *Aphasia.* Psyche Miniatures. Kegan Paul, 1926.
This author is quite convinced that all varieties of Aphasia can be explained on physiological grounds, but produces no convincing reasons. The book is written entirely from the clinical standpoint and is exceedingly valuable ; but the psychology is the old atomic psychology of hypothetical mental units.

3. F. NAVILLE. Mémoires d'un médecin aphasique. *Archives de Psychologie,* Vol. 17, 1919.

4. K. S. LASHLEY. *Brain Mechanisms and Intelligence. Op. cit.,* p. 165.

5. C. J. HERRICK. *Introduction to Neurology,* 4th Ed., pp. 345 foll. W. B. Saunders and Co., 1927.

6. E. MILLER. *Types of Mind and Body.* Kegan Paul, 1926.

7. HALDANE. *Mechanism, Life and Personality,* Ch. 4. Murray, 1921 .

8. C. FOX. Tests of Aphasia. *Brit. Journ. of Psychology,* Vol. 21 (1931).

9. W. VAN WOERKOM. La signification de certains éléments de l'intelligence dans les genèse des troubles aphasiques. *Journ. de Psychologie,* 1921.

10. R. MOURGUE. Disorders of symbolic thinking. *Brit. Journ. of Psychol.* (Medical Section), 1921.

CHAPTER V.—PSYCHOLOGY OF LANGUAGE.

1. A. PICK. *Die agrammatischen Sprachstörungen.* Berlin, 1913.

2. W. STERN. *Psychology of early childhood,* Pt. III. Allen and Unwin, 1924.

3. H. KELLER. *The story of my life.* Hodder and Stoughton, 1903.

4. V. RASMUSSEN. *Child Psychology,* Vol. 1, Ch. 10. Gyldendal, 1920.

5. F. DE SAUSSURE. *Cours de linguistique générale.* Payot. Paris, 2nd Ed., 1922.

6. R. PAGET. *Babel.* Psyche Miniatures. Kegan Paul, 1930.

7. E. W. SCRIPTURE. The nature of verse. *Brit. Journ. of Psychol.,* Vol. 11, 1920.

8. A. SECHEHAYE. Les mirages linguistiques. *Journ. de Psychologie,* 1930.

9. A. M. HOCART. The Psychological interpretation of language. *Brit. Journ. of Psychol.,* Vol. 5, 1912.

10. H. DELACROIX. *Le langage et la pensée.* F. Alcan. Paris, 1924.
A stimulating book on every aspect of language, philosophical, grammatical, psychological, etc.

U

CHAPTER VI.—PSYCHOLOGY OF TEMPERAMENT.

1. HIPPOCRATES. Loeb Classical Library, Vol. I, Introd. W. Heinemann.
2. C. BLOOR. *Temperament*, Ch. 3. Methuen, 1928.
   A good summary of temperaments with some conclusions.
3. C. B. DAVENPORT. Inheritance of temperament. Carnegie Institute. Washington, 1915.
4. L. BERMAN. *The Personal Equation*. Allen and Unwin, 1925.
   See also the same author's *Glands regulating Personality*.
5. W. McDOUGALL. *An outline of Psychology*, Ch. 13. Methuen, 1923.
6. W. B. CANNON. *Bodily changes in Pain, Hunger, etc.* Appleton, 1925.
7. D. WECHSLER. Measurement of Emotional Reactions. *Archives of Psychology*, No. 76. New York, 1925.
8. A. FOUILLÉE. *Tempérament et Caractère*. Felix Alcan, 7th Ed.
9. TH. RIBOT. *Psychologie des Sentiments*. Felix Alcan, 10th Ed. 1917.
   A most penetrating and suggestive study of the emotional life and character.
10. W. JAMES. *Pragmatism*, Ch. 1. Longmans, 1907.
11. C. G. JUNG. *Analytical Psychology*, Ch. 11, 2nd Ed. Baillière, Tindall and Cox, 1917.
    The classification is elaborated in a later book called *Psychological Types*, but the account in the book above is clearer because more concise.
12. E. KRETSCHMER. *Physique and Character*. Int. Lib. Psychol. Kegan Paul, 1925.
13. A. F. SHAND. *Foundations of Character*, Bk. I, Ch. 13. Macmillan, 1914.
14. F. GALTON. *Inquiries into human Faculty*. Everyman's Library. Dent.
15. C. B. DAVENPORT. Violent temper and its inheritance. *Journ. of Nervous and Mental Disease*, 1915.
16. D. W. OATES. An experimental study of temperament. *Brit. Journ. of Psychol.*, Vol. 19, 1928.
    Also R. O. FILTER. An experimental study of character traits. *Journ. of applied psychology*, Vol. 5, 1921.
17. P. G. VERNON. Tests of Temperament. *Brit. Journ. of Psychol.*, Vol. 20, 1930.
18. R. LANGBRIDGE. *Charlotte Brontë*. W. Heinemann, 1929.
    The best brief account of the temperamental relation of body to mind is that given by Dr E. MILLER in *Types of Mind and Body*: a sound and temperate statement of what has been scientifically demonstrated.

CHAPTER VII.—MENTAL ENERGY

1. A. N. WHITEHEAD. *Science and the modern world*, Ch. 1. Camb. Univ. Press, 1926.
2. *Op. cit.*, Ch. 2.
3. W. McDOUGALL. *An Outline of Psychology*, p. 107. Methuen, 1922.

4. C. SPEARMAN. *The Nature of Intelligence*, pp. 5, 131, 346. Macmillan, 1923.
5. K. S. LASHLEY. *Brain Mechanisms*, Ch. 11. Chicago Univ. Press, 1929.
6. H. HEAD. *Aphasia, etc.*, Vol. I, Pt. 3, Ch. 3 ; Pt. 4, Ch. 2. Camb. Univ. Press, 1926.
7. H. C. WARREN. *A history of Association Psychology*, p. 70. Constable, 1921.
8. C. J. HERRICK. *An introduction to neurology*, Ch. 20, 4th Ed. W. B. Saunders, 1927.
9. C. G. JUNG. *Contributions to Analytical Psychology*. Int. Lib. Psychol. Kegan Paul, 1928.
10. J. S. MILL. *System of Logic*, Bk. III, Ch. 20. Longmans, 1896.
11. A. S. EDDINGTON. *Space, Time and Gravitation*, Ch. 9. Camb. Univ. Press, 1921.
12. A. S. EDDINGTON. *Nature of the Physical World*. Camb. Univ. Press, 1928.
13. E. D. ADRIAN. International Congress of Psychology, 1924.
14. C. FOX. *Educational Psychology*, Ch. 12. Int. Lib. Psychol. Kegan Paul, 1928.
15. Fatigue and Work from a 10-hour day in addition. *Journ. of Ed. psychol.*, 1924.
16. Mental Fatigue. *Columbia Univ. Contributions to Education*, No. 54. 1912.
17. E. L. THORNDIKE. *Educational Psychology*, Vol. 3. Columbia Univ. Press, New York, 1913.
18. A. TROLLOPE. *Autobiography*, Ch. 2. World's Classics. Oxford.
19. C. SPEARMAN. *The Abilities of Man*, p. 134. Macmillan.
20. C. S. SHERRINGTON. *Integrative Action of the Nervous System*, Lect. 1. Constable, 1911.
21. I. PAVLOV. *Conditioned Reflexes*, Ch. 13. Oxford Univ. Press.
22. C. FOX. *Practical Psychology*, Ch. 9. Kegan Paul, 1928.
23. A. HILL. *Living Machinery*, Appendix 2. Bell, 1927.

CHAPTER VIII.—INSTINCT AND CUSTOM.

1. W. JAMES. *Text book of psychology*, Ch. 25. Macmillan.
2. E. L. THORNDIKE. *Educational Psychology*, Vol. I. Columbia Univ. Press, New York, 1913.
3. J. DREVER. *Instinct in Man*. Camb. Univ. Press, 1917.
4. W. McDOUGALL. *Outline of Psychology*, Ch. 4. Methuen.
5. C. M. DOUGHTY. *Travels in Arabia Deserta*, Vol. 1, Ch. 8, p. 240. Camb. Univ. Press, 1888.
6. J. B. WATSON. *Psychology from the standpoint of a behaviourist*. Lippincott, 1919.
7. A. M. CARR-SAUNDERS. *The population problem*. Oxford Univ. Press, 1922.
   My quotation from Glotz is taken from this learned book.
8. A. M. CARR-SAUNDERS. *Op. cit.*, p. 215 and Ch. XI.

9. C. W. Margold. *Sex Freedom and Social Control.* Univ. of Chicago Press, 1926.

10. *Op. cit.*, Ch. 3.

11. G. C. Allen. *Modern Japan.* Allen and Unwin, 1928.

12. B. Russell. *Marriage and Morals*, Ch. 2. Allen and Unwin, 1929.

13. C. F. Burk. Pedagogical Seminary, Vol. 7, pp. 179–207.

14. Lehman and Witly. Tendency to collect and hoard. *Psychol. Review*, Vol. 34, 1927.

15. Heidbreder. Thinking as an instinct. *Psychol. Review*, Vol. 33, 1926.

16. G. R. de Beer. *Embryology and Evolution*, Ch. 2. Oxford Univ. Press, 1930.

17. J. M. Fletcher. An old solution of the new problem of instinct. *Psychol. Review*, Vol. 36, 1929.

18. C. S. Myers. *Experimental Psychology*, 2nd Ed., p. 136. Camb. Univ. Press, 1911.

19. J. C. Field. Faculty Psychology and Instinct Psychology. *Mind*, July 1921.

20. J. Dewey. *Human Nature and Conduct*, Pt. 2, Ch. 6. Allen and Unwin, 1922.
   The best treatise on instinct ever written.

21. B. Russell. *On Education.* Allen and Unwin, 1926.

22. C. W. Valentine. Innate bases of Fear. *Journ. of Genetic Psychology*, Vol. 37, 1930.

23. C. Fox. *Educational Psychology*, Ch. 5. Int. Lib. Psychol. Kegan Paul, 1928.
   I have attempted to shew in this book that habits have impulsive power.

CHAPTER IX.—A GREAT ILLUSION.

1. G. F. Stout. *Manual of Psychology*, 4th Ed., Bk. 1, Ch. 2. W. B. Clive, 1929.

2. F. Galton. *Inquiry into human faculty.* Everyman Series. Dent·

3. E. R. Jaensch. *Eidetic Imagery.* Int. Lib. Psychol. Kegan Paul.

4. G. Dawes Hicks. On the Nature of Images. *Brit. Journ. of Psychol.*, Vol. 15, 1924.

5. G. Berkeley. *Principles of Human Knowledge*, Pt. III. Everyman Series. Dent.

6. J. Drever. *Instinct in Man*, Ch. 6 and Appendix 1. Camb. Univ. Press, 1917.

7. E. Miller. The affective nature of illusion and hallucination. *Journ. of Neurology and Psychopathology*, Vol. 8, 1927.

8. A. L. Wigan. *Duality of the Mind*, Ch. 9, p. 84. Longmans, 1844.

9. E. Bernard-Leroy. *L'Illusion de fausse reconnaissance.* F. Alcan (Paris), 1898.

10. G. H. Lewes. *Problems of life and mind*, 3rd Series, Problem 2, 1879.

11. Quoted by E. Bernard-Leroy. *Op. cit.*, Ch. 8.

12. Révész and Hazenwinkel. Didactic value of lantern slides and films. *Brit. Journ. of Psychol.*, Vol. 15, 1924.
13. S. Alexander. Creative Process in the artist's mind. *Brit. Journ. of Psychol.*, Vol. 17, 1927.
14. A. Trollope. *Autobiography*, Chs. 3 and 8. World's Classics. Oxford.
15. J. W. Dunne. *An Experiment with Time*, Ch. 12, 2nd Ed. A. and C. Black, 1929.

CHAPTER X.—EDUCATIONAL PSYCHOLOGY.

1. C. Fox. *Educational Psychology*, 2nd Ed. Int. Lib. Psychol. Kegan Paul, 1928.
2. Schools Inquiry Commission Report, Vol. 1, Ch. 1, 1868.
   This whole chapter is worth reading as it expresses the enlightened view of those who approved the doctrine at that period when it dominated education.
3. E. L. Thorndike and R. S. Woodworth. Influence of Improvement in one mental function, etc. *Psy. Review*, Vol. 8.
4. Langdon and Yates. An exp. investigation into transfer of training. *Brit. Journ. of Psychol.*, Vol. 18, 1928.
5. E. L. Thorndike. *Educational Psychology*, Vol. 2. Columbia Univ. Press, New York.
6. C. V. D. Hadley. Transfer experiments with guinea-pigs. *Brit. Journ. of Psychol.*, Vol. 18, 1928.
7. W. Köhler. *Mentality of Apes*. Int. Lib. Psychol. Kegan Paul, 1925.
8. H. Woodrow. Effect of type of training upon transference. *Journ. of Educ. Psychology*, Vol. 18, 1927.
9. A. N. Whitehead. *Introduction to Mathematics*, Ch. 1. Home Univ. Library.
10. G. P. Meredith. Consciousness of method as a means of transfer of training. *Forum of Educ.*, Vol. 5, 1927.
11. T. H. Pear. The nature of skill. *Journ. of Industrial Psychol.*, Vol. 4, 1928.
12. J. Ward. *The Realm of Ends*, p. 449. Camb. Univ. Press, 1911.

CHAPTER XI.—MIND MATTER AND PHILOSOPHERS.

1. J. G. Frazer. *Taboo*. Macmillan, 1911.
2. P. Janet and G. Séailles. *History of the Problems of Philosophy*, Pt. III. Macmillan, 1902.
   The opinions of the ancient and some modern philosophers are collected in a convenient form.
3. Haldane and Ross. *Philosophical Works of Descartes*. Camb. Univ. Press, 1911.
4. W. D. Ross. *Aristotle's Metaphysics*, Introd., p. cxliii. Oxford Univ. Press, 1924.
5. R. D. Hicks. *Aristotle: de Anima*, Introduction. Camb. Univ. Press, 1907.
6. J. Ward. *Realm of Ends*, Note III. Camb. Univ. Press, 1911.

7. W. James. *Principles of Psychology*, Vol. 1, Ch. X. Macmillan.
8. C. Lloyd Morgan. *Emergent Evolution*. Williams and Norgate, 1923.
9. R. Latta. *Leibniz, the Monadology*, Introduction. Oxford Univ. Press, 1898.
10. H. S. Jennings. *Biological basis of human nature*. Faber and Faber, 1930.
11. A. S. Eddington. *Nature of the physical world*. Camb. Univ. Press, 1928.
12. B. Russell. *Outline of Philosophy*. Allen and Unwin, 1927.
13. A. N. Whitehead. *Science and the Modern World*. Camb. Univ. Press, 1926.

CHAPTER XII.—MIND AND BODY.

1. G. F. Stout. *Manual of Psychology*, Ch. 3, 4th Ed. Clive, 1929.
2. J. F. Dashiell. Is the Cerebrum the seat of thinking. *Psychol. Review*, Vol. 33, 1926.
   A. D. Ritchie. Relations of Mental and Physical Processes. *Mind*, Vol. 40, 1931.
3. L. Carmichael. (a) Development of behaviour in vertebrates, etc. *Psychol. Review*, Vol. 33, 1926.
   (b) A further study of behaviour of vertebrates, etc. *Psychol. Review*, Vol. 34, 1927.
4. A. S. Eddington. *Nature of the Physical World*, Ch. 5. Camb. Univ. Press, 1928.
5. J. Ward. *Psychological Principles*, Ch. 8. Camb. Univ. Press, 1918.
6. K. S. Lashley. Basic Neural Mechanisms, etc. *Psychol. Review*. Vol. 7, 1930.
7. C. Fox. Tests of Aphasia. *Brit. Journ. of Psychol.*, Vol. 21, 1931.
8. A. Wohlgemuth. The conditioned reflex, etc. *Journ. of Mental Science*, Oct. 1930.
9. H. Schlosberg. Study of the conditioned patellar reflex. *Journ. of Exp. Psychol.*, Vol. 11, 1928.
10. W. Lankes. Perseveration. *Brit. Journ. of Psychol.*, Vol. 7, 1915.
11. Winsor and Bayne. Unconditioned salivary response in man. *Amer. Journ. of Psychol.*, Vol. 41, 1929.
12. C. Lloyd Morgan. *Emergent Evolution*. Williams and Norgate 1923.
13. S. Butler. *Life and Habit*. Fifield.
14. E. P. Bowne. *Metaphysics*. Quoted in James' *Principles*, Vol. 1, p. 219.
15. A. N. Whitehead. *Science and the Modern World*, Ch. 9. Camb. Univ. Press.
16. W. E. Johnson. *Logic*, Pt. 3, Ch. 8. Camb. Univ. Press, 1924.
17. G. P. Thomson. *The Atom*, Ch. 15. Home Univ. Library. Thornton and Butterworth.
18. Kant. *Fundamental Principles of Metaphysics of Ethics*, Par. 88. Translated by Abbott. Longmans, 1907.
19. H. G. Wyatt. *Psychology of Intelligence and Will*, Pt. III. Int. Lib. Psychol. Kegan Paul, 1930.

INDEX

ACT of apprehension, analysis of, 209
Action current, in nerves, 27
Adrenal glands, function of, 133
Adrian, E. D., ' all or none ' rule, 28 ; cause of sensation, 36 ; on mental energy, 163
Adult's *v.* children's speech, 112
Agnosia, 83
Agraphia, 85
Aleatory instinct, 192
Alexander, S., on emergent evolution, 251 ; on artistic creation 220
' All or none ' rule, 28
Allen, G. C., on Japanese sex relations, 188
Analogy, dangers of, 175 ; *J. S. Mill* on, 160
Anarthria, 82
Anaxagoras, on mind and matter, 241
Aphasia, a psychological defect, 2 ; its true nature, 102 ; its varieties, 87
Aphasic paradoxes, 79
Appearance and reality, 298
Appetites, their nature, 198
Apraxia, 82
Area striata and vision, 61
Aristotle, active and passive intellect, 245 ; on matter and form, 242, 244
' Association fibres,' 18 ; and habit, 69
Association of ideas, by emotion, 217 ; law of, 17
Association *v.* intelligence, 107
Asthenic physique, 141
Athletic fatigue, 173 ; physique, 141
Atomic structure, 256
Attention, active and passive, 43 ; and fatigue, 174 ; essential for conditioned reflex, 38 ; not a faculty, 14 ; organ of, 14

Bacon on Studies, 226
Ball, J., on reflexes, 75

Bayne and *Winsor*, conditioned reflex, 282
Behaviourism, 264, 286
Bergson, H., his method, 246
Berkeley, on sensations, 208 ; perception of distance, 42
Berman, L., glands regulating temperament, 132
Bernard-Leroy, E., on déjà vu, 215
Betting, as an instinct, 192
Boirac, E., on déjà vu, 218
Bowne, E. P., on thought transference, 286
Brain functions, how studied, 55 ; interconnected, 97
Broad, C. D., on nerve physiology, 63
Broca, on aphasia, 78
Broca's convolution, 78
Brown, T., law of association, 158
Burk, C. F., instinct of collecting, 190
Butler, S., *Life and habit*, 180 ; on evolution, 285

Cannon, W. B., bodily changes in emotion, 135
Carmichael, L., maturation of function, 266
Carr-Saunders, A. M., on infanticide, 184 ; *Population problem*, 191
Cerebral cortex, and consciousness, 263 ; and mental action, 11 ; functions of, 57, 94
Cerebral lesions, in monkeys, 65
Children's *v.* adult's speech, 112
Chronaxy, 31 ; and temperament, 150
Cognition, analysis of, 209
Conception *v.* perception, 272
Conceptual *v.* perceptual time, 269
Conditioned reflex, 37, 279 ; a misnomer, 75 ; equivalent to association, 45 ; in man, 42 ; origin of

name, 39; conditions for, 43; in man, 280
Conscious action, criterion of, 21
Conventional v. inborn in speech, 113
Co-ordination centres, 15
Correspondence of mind and brain, 15, 25; of mind and body, 267; of mental and physical, 270
Cowper, quoted, 117
Criteria for instincts, 177
Curiosity, instinct of, 189
Cyclothymic temperament, 142

Dashiell, J. F., localization of thought, 265
Davenport, C. B., inheritance of temper, 145
Dawes Hicks, G., analysis of cognition, 209; on images, 208
Death, theory of, 240
de Beer, G. R., structure and function, 194
Déjà vu, 214
Delacroix, H., on emotional expression, 115; on language values, 128
Dementia præcox, 141
Democritus, 241
de Saussure, F., Cours de Linguistique générale, 113; quoted, 122
Descartes, on animal spirits, 8; on mind and body, 246; on memory, 9; on vital functions, 8; sunders mind and matter, 243
Determinism and calculability, 295
Dewey, J., Human nature and conduct, 197; on appetites, 198; on instincts, 202
Diagrams, on the brain, 80
Diaschisis, 98
Dickens, on false recognition, 214
Dr Johnson, refutation of Berkeley, 261
Doughty, C. M., Beduin affections, 181; *Travels in Arabia Deserta*, 189
Downey, will-temperament tests, 148
Dreams, 206; true interpretation of, 109
Drever, J., analysis of perception, 210; on instinct, 180
Dunne, J. W., Experiment with time, 216

Economic man, 51

Eddington, A. S., nature of physics, 260; on atomic space, 256; on physics, 10; on Time, 268
Educational values, 232
Eidetic images, 206
Einstein, on gravitation, 163
Elliot Smith, G., on organ of attention, 13; on pugnacious instinct, 191
Embryo, development of, 251
Emergence, of new self, 297
Emergent evolution, 22, 283
Emotional expression, in language, 114
Emotions and instincts, 178
Empathy, 212
Empedocles, on elements, 130
Endocrine glands and temperament, 132
Endurance, of time, 269
Energy, modern conception of, 163
Energy fund, experiments on, 164
Entropy, 268; clocks, 270; psychical, 162
Epistemology, inadequate for mind, 6; of language, 105
Equipotentiality, of cortical areas, 57; of function, 102
Extensity, in space perception, 276
Extraverts, 140

Faculty of attention, objection to, 14
False recognition, 214
Fatigue, and attention, 174; and mental energy, 153; experiment by *C. Fox*, 171; in athletes, 173; measured by variability, 172
Fears, diversity of, 200; how aroused, 199
Field, J. C., on faculty psychology, 197
Films v. lantern slides, 219
Florence Nightingale, her capacity for work, 165
Fortescue, Earl, on mental training, 226
Fouillée, character and temperament, 145; on temperament, 137
Fox, C., Educational psychology, 164, 227, 236; experiment on fatigue, 171
Franz, S. I., on reflexes, 67; maze experiments, 56
Frazer, J. G., savage reasoning, 240
Freedom, as emergent, 297; as experienced, 298

Freedom of will, 294 ; *Kant* on, 296
Freud, S., mythical censor, 109
Function, independent of structure, 97
Fund of energy, experiments on, 164

Galen, on temperament, 130
Gall, on cerebral localisation, 78
Galton, F., on energy, 152 ; on inheritance in twins, 145 ; on mental images, 205, 213
Genesis, on universal language, 104
Gestalt psychology, 235
Glotz, on infanticide, 183
Grimm, phonetic law, 127
Guinea-pigs, training of, 229
Guthrie, E. R., on conditioned reflex, 45

HABIT, and association fibres, 69 ; growth of, 285 ; impulsive power of, 201
Haldane, on nervous function, 100 ; on stimulus and response, 39
Hallucinations, origin of, 206 ; *v.* images, 206 ; varieties of, 213
Hartley, law of association, 158 ; on sensations and images, 53 ; *Observations on Man*, 52
Head, Henry, aphasia, 77, 279 ; emotion and aphasia, 93 ; nervous function, 157 ; on nervous action, 23 ; on symbolic expression, 87 ; on 'vigilance,' 16 ; tests of aphasia, 100
Heredity and environment, 195, 266
Herrick, C. J., on association of ideas, 158
Hippocrates, on temperament, 130
Hitzig, on visual area, 61
Hocart, A. M., on Fijian language, 125
Homer, on the soul, 240
Hughlings-Jackson, on aphasia, 78 ; on propositions, 80
Human nature, changeable, 201
Hypokinetic temperament, 131

IDEALS, power of, 236
Illusion, character of, 203 ; of moving train, 222 ; Müller-Lyer's, 222; of false recognition, 214
Images, of a dog, 273 ; 'free' and 'tied,' 272 ; pre-existence of, 35 ;

their antics, 241 ; *v.* sensations, 207
Imitation, its spontaneity, 109
Immortality of the soul, 300
Impressions, fusion of, 275
Infanticide, prevalence of, 183
Inhibition, conditions of, 46 ; learning by, 47
Inspiration, 239
Instinct, of betting, 192 ; of collecting, 190 ; of curiosity, 189 ; of thinking, 192 ; maternal, 182 ; parental, 181
Instincts, and emotions, 178 ; enumeration of, 178 ; not innate, 4
Instrumental relation, 248
Intelligence *v.* association, 107
Interactionism, assumptions of, 261
Introverts, 140
Invention of words, by children, 108

Jaensch, E. R., on eidetic images, 206
James, W., beginning of experience, 271 ; criteria of instincts, 177 ; energies of men, 168 ; enumeration of instincts, 178 ; on brain functions, 53 ; on mind and body, 248 ; stream of consciousness, 84 ; temperamental types, 138
James-Lange, theory of emotions, 135, 245
Japanese, sex customs of, 187
Jennings, H. S., embryonic development, 252
Joan of Arc, 206
Johnson, W. E., on one-to-one correspondence, 62 ; on volition, 293 ; the continuant, 242
Jung, C. G., on libido, 169 ; on psychical energy, 159, 161 ; temperamental types, 139

Kant, freedom of will, 296 ; on temperament, 131
Keller, Helen, discovery of naming, 111
Kinnier Wilson, S. A., on aphasia, 86, 93
Köhler, W., mentality of apes, 230
Kraepelin, on false recognition, 215; types of insanity, 141
Kretschmer, E., cyclothymes and schizothymes, 143 ; *Physique and character*, 141

Lalande, on déjà vu, 215
Langbridge, R., on personality, 151
Language, a material-spiritual unity, 128 ; a social institution, 123 ; and mentality, 124 ; and thought, 121 ; development, in children, 106 ; functions of, 94 ; entirely a thought product, 129 ; mutilation of, 109
Lankes, W., on perseveration, 282
Lantern slides v. films, 219
Lapicque, L., on chronaxy, 31
Lashley, K. S., functions of cortex, 58 ; maze experiments, 56 ; on habit-formation, 68, 76 ; on habit-mechanisms, 64 ; on nervous energy, 156 ; on one-to-one correspondence, 277 ; on reflexes, 75 ; on restitution of function, 70
Law of association, equivalent to conditioned reflex, 45
Learning, by inhibition, 47 ; by substituting stimuli, 42
Leibniz, monadology, 253 ; on dispositions, 180 ; on innate dispositions, 176 ; on matter, 243 ; on organism, 6 ; unity of universe, 251
Lewes, G. H., on déjà vu, 218
Liberal education, 232
Libido, or mental energy, 161
Lillie, R. S., ' impulses ' in wires, 33
Linguistic values, 120
Living tissue, essential to sensation, 33
Living v. dead tissue, 262
Lloyd Morgan, C., on emergent evolution, 251, 283
Localization, of function, 57, 263 ; a misnomer, 99 ; reasons for, 84 ; of thinking, 265
Locke, J., on innate ideas, 288 ; on mental discipline, 225 ; tabula rasa, 176
Loss of function, cause of, 92

Malinowski, B., Trobriand Islanders, 186
Manic-depressive insanity, 141
Margold, C. W., on sexual conduct, 185
Marie, P., on aphasia, 82
Marshall Hall, on reflex action, 72, 279
Matter and Mind v. Body and Mind, 5
Matter, nature of, 257 ; organic view of, 258

' Maze ' experiments, 56
McDougall, W., definition of instinct, 179 ; fund of energy, 155 ; glands regulating temperament, 134 ; list of instincts, 179
Meditation, Descartes', 243
Memories, not stored up, 19
Memory, and brain, 19 ; *Descartes* on, 9
Mental, capacity, how measured, 235 ; discipline, 224 ; dispositions, their nature, 196 ; energy, 193 ; energy distinct from nervous, 3 ; energy and fatigue, 153 ; events, and neural events, 62 ; factors, in bodily activity, 67 ; fatigue and energy, 3 ; images and the brain, 4 ; images, distinguished from concepts, 117 ; images, reality of, 223 ; structure, 195 ; training, method of investigation, 226 ; training, by science, 233
Meynert's diagrams, 19
Mill, J. S., on analogy, 160
Miller, E., on hallucinations, 214 ; on nervous function, 99
Mind, ambiguity of, 293 ; as ego, 293 ; as psychoplasm, 293 ; mirrors brain, 10
Mind-body relation, unique, 255, 290 ; parts of, 292 ; terms of, 7 ; four terms, 291
Mind-body, a unique unity, 103
Minkowski, on visual area, 61
Mixed temperaments, 147
Monadology, 253
' Motor area,' in brain, 13 ; discovery of, 81 ; variability of, 23
Motor cortex, very variable, 91
Mourgue, R., nature of aphasia, 102
Moving train illusion, 203
Mrs Trollope, capacity for work, 167
Müller-Lyer illusion, 222
Munk, H., discovers visual area, 81
Myers, C. S., on perseveration, 196

NATIONAL characters, 138
Nerve centres, 15 ; how determined, 90 ; not fixed, 98
Nerve impulses, 27, 247
Nerves and sensation, 26
Nervous, action, 278
Neural events, and mental events, 62
Neurology, postulates of, 1
Nominal aphasia, 88

Oates, D. W., experiment on temperament, 148
Occipital lobes and vision, 60
Ogden, on reflexes, 67
On Man, Descartes, 8
One-to-one correspondence, 62, 270
Oral words, elements of, 116
Organic sensations, 287
Organic life, its nature, 264
Organization, a teleological concept, 270
Others' minds, knowledge of, 286

Paget, Sir R., origin of speech, 113
Parallelism, assumptions of, 261
Parental instinct, 181
Parmenides, 241
' Pathways,' or ' traces ' in nerves, 54
Pavlov, J. P., conditioned reflexes, 37 ; fatigue and rhythm, 170 ; functions of brain, 38 ; on sleep, 50 ; physiology of attention, 46
Pear, T. H., on habits, 236
Perception, analysis of, 210
Perception *v.* conception, 272
Perseveration, 196, 281
Physics, and symbolism, 10 ; the science of symbols, 260
Physiological postulates, 11
Physiological *v.* real animal, 51
Physiology of *Descartes*, 9
Pick, A., structure of language, 105
Piéron, H., on co-ordination centres, 15
Plato, Republic, 224
Platonic Ideas, 238
Pre-established harmony, 254
Presentations, defined, 300
Protensity, in time perception, 274
Psycho-analysis, 49 ; and images, 34
Psycho-galvanic reflex, 136
Psychological process *v.* physiological, 86
Psycho-physical parallelism, 267
Psychoplasm, 293
Pyknic physique, 141
Pythagoreans, 241

REASONING, of savages, 240
Reflex action, its fatality, 20 ; its parts, 21 ; and voluntary actions, 74 ; inborn, 37 ; involves mental factors, 67
Reflex theory, 71
Repetitive work, 238

Restitution of function, 24, 70
Ribot, T., on character, 144 ; on personalities, 138
Richerand, on temperament, 131
Ritchie, A. D., localization of function, 265
Rivers, W. H., on claustrophobia, 161
Russell, B., appearances constitute reality, 289 ; fear in children, 199 ; nature of matter, 257 ; on mathematics, 237 ; on sex instinct, 189

SALIVARY reflex, 282
Saloz, Dr, on aphasia, 95
Savage languages, characters of, 126
Schizothymic temperament, 142
Schools Inquiry Commission on mental training, 225
Scripture, E. W., analysis of spoken words, 118
Sechehaye, A., on language, 124
Self-determination, 294
Semantic aphasia, 88
Sensation and nerves, 26
Sensations, knowledge of, 293 ; origin of inexplicable, 36 ; theory of, 287 ; *v.* images, 207
Sense-data, abstractions, 284
Sensing, act of, 211
Sensory areas in brain, 12
Sex practices, diversity of, 186
Sexual instinct, 185
Shakespeare, appreciation of, 291
Shand, A. F., Foundations of character, 147 ; on temperament, 143
Sherrington, C. S., on fatigue, 170
Signalling stimuli, 38
Significance *v.* value in words, 120
Sleep, physiology of, 49
Souls, kinds of, 242
Space perception, 276
Spearman, C., fund of energy, 155 ; on fatigue, 168
Speech development, stages of, 111
Speech, entirely psychical, 86
Spinoza, mind and matter, 243 ; on world-soul, 251 ; physical and psychical, 285 ; unity of mind and body, 250
Spoken *v.* written language, 113
Stern, W., speech in children, 107
' Stimulus,' ambiguity of term, 39 ; meaning of, 230
Stout, G. F., function of cerebral cortex, 263 ; images *v.* impressions, 204 ; on sensation, 26

Strachey, Lytton, Eminent Victorians, 165
Structure *v.* function, 194
Subjective activity, 5
Subjective insight, into mind, 290
Subject-object relation, 254
Suppression, nervous, 49
Symbolism, and physics, 10, 260 ; analysed, 116 ; in speech, 113
Syntactical aphasia, 88

Telegraphist's cramp, 281
Temperament, an artistic concept, 3, 151 ; in animals, 50 ; *v.* temper, 146
Temperamental relation, meaning of, 130
Temperaments are adjectives, 149
Temporal signs, 275
The soul, immortality of, 300
Thermo-dynamics, second law of, 268
Thomas Bertrand, South Arabia, 126 ; time-sense of Arabs, 274
Thomson, G. P., on determinism, 295
Thorndike, E. L., enumeration of instincts, 178 ; on fatigue, 165, 170 ; on mental training, 227, 228
Thought and language, 122
Thurstone, L. L., on ' stimulus,' 41
Thyroid gland, function of, 133
Time perception, direction in, 274
Transcendental self, 298
Trollope, Anthony, Autobiography, 167, 221

Valentine, C. W., on fear, 200
Values, appreciation of, 298 ; extra-psychological, 237
van Woerkom, W., spatial disability in aphasics, 101
Velasquez, Spanish Admiral, 220
Verbal aphasia, 87

Vernon, P. E., on temperament, 150
Vesalius, on mental functions, 53
Vicarious functioning in cerebrum, 69
' Vigilance ' of nerves, 17
Vision and occipital lobes, 60
' Visual area ' of cortex, 62 ; discovery of, 81
Vital activity, rhythmical, 174
Volition, 293

Ward, J., on mind and body, 254 ; on the realm of ends, 238 ; on time perception, 276
Watson, J. B., on fear, 199 ; on instinct, 54 ; on maternal behaviour, 182
Wave mechanics, 256, 257
Wechsler, D., on psycho-galvanic reflex, 136
Westermarck, on sexual conduct, 187
Whistler, on artistic subjects, 219
Whitehead, A. N., mathematical education, 232 ; matter as organic, 258, 262 ; on organism, 6 ; on scientific concepts, 153 ; perception of minds, 289
Wigan, A. L., Duality of the Mind, 214 ; on cerebral lag, 216
Will, freedom of, 294
Winsor and *Bayne,* conditioned reflex, 282
Wohlgemuth, A., on conditioned reflex, 279
Woodrow, H., on memory training, 231
Woodworth, R. S., on mental training, 227
Word-identity, 119
Word images, not stored, 36
Word values, 80, 120
Words, complexity of significance, 123 ; not separate, 118
Writer's cramp, 281
Wyatt, H. G., on volition, 298